Care of People with Diabetes:
A Manual of Nursing Practice

Other books of interest:

The Royal Marsden Hospital Manual of Clinical Nursing Procedures
A. Phylip Pritchard and Jane Mallett
0 632 03387 8

Handbook of Diabetes
G. Williams and J. C. Pickup
0 632 02888 2

Diabetes and its Management
Fourth Edition
P. J. Watkins, P. L. Drury and K. W. Taylor
0 632 02692 8

Health Promotion – Concepts and Practice
A. Dines and A. Cribb
0 632 03543 9

Expanding the Role of the Nurse – The Scope of Professional Practice
G. Hunt and P. Wainwright
0 632 03604 4

The Care of Wounds – A Guide for Nurses
C. Dealey
0 632 03864 0

Care of People with Diabetes:
A Manual of Nursing Practice

Trisha Dunning
RN, RM, IW, Grad Dip Health Ed, MEd, FRCNA
Clinical Nurse Consultant
Diabetes Education, St Vincent's Hospital
Melbourne, Australia

OXFORD

BLACKWELL SCIENTIFIC PUBLICATIONS

LONDON EDINBURGH BOSTON

MELBOURNE PARIS BERLIN VIENNA

© 1994 by
Blackwell Scientific Publications
Editorial Offices:
Osney Mead, Oxford OX2 0EL
25 John Street, London WC1N 2BL
23 Ainslie Place, Edinburgh EH3 6AJ
238 Main Street, Cambridge,
    Massachusetts 02142, USA
54 University Street, Carlton,
    Victoria 3053, Australia

Other Editorial Offices:
Librairie Arnette SA
1, rue de Lille
75007 Paris
France

Blackwell Wissenschafts-Verlag GmbH
Düsseldorfer Str. 38
D-10707 Berlin
Germany

Blackwell MZV
Feldgasse 13
A-1238 Wien
Austria

First published 1994

Set by DP Photosetting, Aylesbury, Bucks
Printed and bound in Great Britain by
Hartnolls Ltd, Bodmin, Cornwall

DISTRIBUTORS
Marston Book Services Ltd
PO Box 87
Oxford OX2 0DT
(*Orders*: Tel: 0865 791155
        Fax: 0865 791927
        Telex: 837515

USA
Blackwell Scientific Publications, Inc.
238 Main Street
Cambridge, MA 02142
(*Orders*: Tel: 800 759-6102
            617 876-7000)

Canada
Times Mirror Professional Publishing, Ltd
130 Flaska Drive
Markham, Ontario L6G 1B8
(*Orders*: Tel: 800 268-4178
            416 470-6739)

Australia
Blackwell Scientific Publications Pty Ltd
54 University Street,
Carlton, Victoria 3053
(*Orders*: Tel: 03 347-5552)

British Library
Cataloguing in Publication Data
A Catalogue record for this book is available from the
British Library

ISBN 0–632–03876–4

Library of Congress
Cataloging in Publication Data
Dunning, Trisha.
    Care of people with diabetes: a manual of nursing
practice/Trisha Dunning.
    p.   cm.
    Includes bibliographical references and index.
    ISBN 0–632–03876–4
    1. Diabetes—Nursing. I. Title.
    [DNLM: 1. Diabetes Mellitus—nursing—
handbooks.   WY 39 D924c 1994]
RC660.D785   1994
610.73′69—dc20
DNLM/DLC
for Library of Congress   93-46697
                                                CIP

Dedication

This book is dedicated to all people with diabetes
who may one day need to be in
hospital, and to all nurses who care for them.

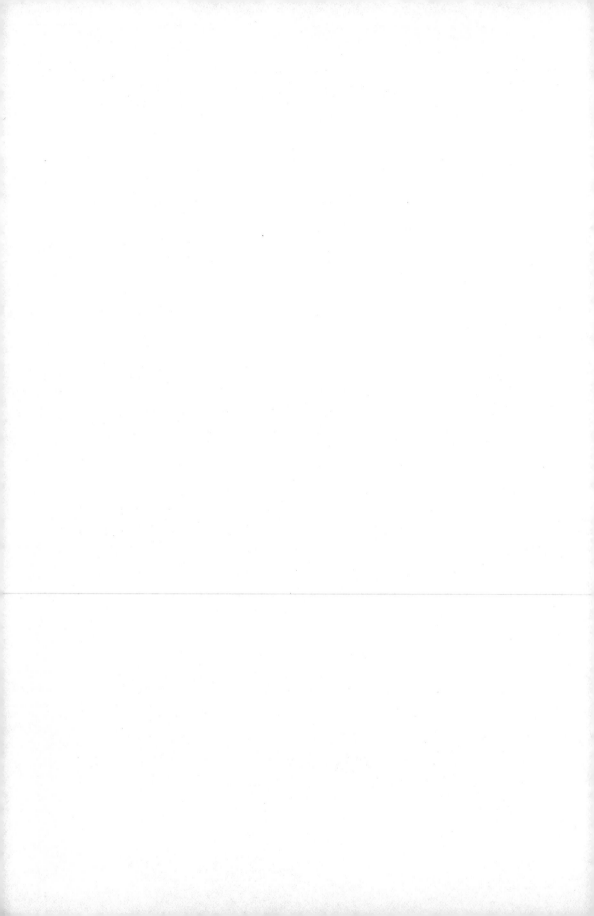

Contents

Foreword

Since the discovery of insulin in 1921–2, the progress of diabetes care has been marked not only by extensive research and development in the field of medicine, but also in pharmacology, biochemistry, technology and information systems. As the twenty-first century approaches, people with diabetes and those caring for them have the opportunity to work together, with all the advantages that modern health care can provide. Despite all this, however, living with diabetes is not easy. There remains much fear about this disease and many myths and misconceptions surrounding the condition, all of which affect nursing and medical care provided by the many health care professionals involved during the lifetime of a person with diabetes.

In recognition of the growing global problem of diabetes, the forty-second World Health Assembly adopted in May 1989 a resolution (WHA 42.36) on the prevention and control of diabetes. This resolution invited Member States to assess the national importance of diabetes, to implement population based measures for its prevention and control, and to 'share opportunities for training and further education'.

It has been said that 'diabetes is an easy disease to treat badly'. On admission to hospital the person with diabetes is disadvantaged and often in the hands of professionals with many skills but little knowledge of diabetes and its management. *Care of People with Diabetes* will be especially welcome for them. It is practical, thoughtful and delightfully written by an experienced clinical nurse specialist with extensive knowledge of diabetes care. Here, surely, is a perfect example of an opportunity taken to 'share training and further education' and this book should be an *essential* source of up-to-date information for nurses, doctors and many others in clinical practice.

Mary MacKinnon, *MMED, Sci, RGN*
Diabetes Nurse Specialist Co-ordinator
Course Teacher, Sheffield and North Trent
College of Nursing and Midwifery
Member The St Vincent Joint Task Force for Diabetes, UK

Preface

Background

Teaching nursing staff and other health professionals is an important part of my role as a diabetes educator in an acute care teaching hospital. A chance remark, 'Why don't you publish these overhead projections?' following one lecture, sowed the seed which was to eventually become this book: *Care of People with Diabetes: A Manual of Nursing Practice*.

The book has been three years in the writing, but is based on ten years' experience as a Clinical Nurse Consultant in diabetes education and over 20 years' experience as a Registered Nurse. Some of the information has been gleaned from the patients themselves.

I have chosen to refer to people with diabetes in contact with a health care agency as 'patients'. The word 'patient' suggests to me the caring relationship that is nursing, in a way that 'client' and 'customer' do not.

Diabetes mellitus is a chronic disease affecting a significant number of people worldwide, although ethnic susceptibility varies between races. The acute short-term metabolic disturbance, and the long-term complications of diabetes, account for a significant number of hospital admissions requiring specialized knowledge and nursing care.

Nurses have a responsibility to ensure they have adequate knowledge in order to provide competent care. A wide literature search failed to identify adequate documentation of the specific nursing care of people with diabetes, although the medical aspects are covered in detail. This Manual attempts to address the apparent lack of documentation. The aim was to formulate *Care of People with Diabetes: A Manual of Nursing Practice* (The Manual), to be used as a self-directed learning resource and ready reference text in the clinical setting.

The draft Manual was evaluated in two wards and the domiciliary service of an acute care university teaching hospital. Endocrinologists, diabetes educators and specialist practitioners read the text to ensure that the information is accurate. The consensus of opinion was that the contents are accurate, easily understood and will be a useful resource in the clinical areas. There was a self-reported increase in knowledge about diabetic nursing care by all health professionals who evaluated the material.

It is my hope that this Manual will contribute to the body of nursing knowledge about diabetes, and that it will be of assistance to nurses (and other health professionals) involved in the care of people with diabetes. I have endeavoured to make the information general and applicable to all nurses; I hope each person who reads the Manual will find something of value.

Using the Manual

'The nurse, more than any other member of the health team, is the person who interprets to the patient the care he must take of himself and his family. Her belief in the comprehensiveness of adequate care will influence the scope of her care beyond the treatment prescribed by the physician.'

(Henderson, 1966)

Nursing is both an art and a science whose essence is caring. Nurses have a responsibility (with other health professionals) for planning, implementing and evaluating the care given to patients under their care. Nurses function in a variety of settings and the components of the nurse's role varies according to the setting (hospital, community health centres, city or remote areas).

Nursing care is distinct from medical care, but complements the medical plan. Some nursing actions are dictated by the medical orders, others are the basis on which the medical orders are formulated. It is of the utmost importance, then, that nurses have adequate knowledge about disease processes and their effect on individuals in order to provide optimal care.

People who have had diabetes for some time are often aware of omissions and poorly performed procedures relating to their care in hospital. In the case of diabetics, this is particularly true of blood glucose testing and insulin administration. A lack of trust in the staff, considerable anxiety and confusion about the correct method can result if ward staff practice is not consistent with that of the diabetes education team.

This Manual has been designed as a quick reference source for specific nursing actions needed in the care of people with diabetes mellitus in hospital. It is designed for use at the bedside, as revision notes for examinations and for use at undergraduate level. It may also assist in the nursing assessment of diabetic patients aiding the formulation of appropriate nursing care plans, provided the care required for other concurrent disease processes is included in the plan. A list of key points is given at the beginning of each chapter. Important points are highlighted in the text with a rule above and below the information.

In addition to the reference material for nursing staff and patients (Appendixes B and C, respectively), most chapters in this manual are accompanied by a list of recommended reading to assist in self-directed learning and the acquisition of further knowledge. The texts cited are all readily available. Chapters are cross-referenced where appropriate. The pathophysiology and medical management of diabetes is discussed only briefly; a sample of the texts available dealing with these topics is given at the beginning of Appendix B.

The care outlined in this Manual does not negate the provision of basic general nursing care as indicated by the presenting condition, but focuses on the specific and extra needs of people with diabetes when they are admitted to hospital. The presence of diabetes will have physiological effects on the presenting condition if diabetes is not adequately controlled. Most of the care described is based on independent nursing actions, however, some will have a collaborative basis.

The procedure and policies of the employing institution should be followed. This manual does not replace these documents.

Further reading

Cohen, H. (1981) *The Nurse's Quest for a Professional Identity*. Addison Wesley, Menlo Park, California.
Henderson, V. (1966) *The Nature of Nursing*. Macmillan, New York.

Acknowledgements

I would like to acknowledge the support and encouragement received from many people during the writing of this book; in particular Professor Marjory Martin for her constructive comments and belief in my ability to succeed.

I would like to thank Drs Frank Alford and Glenn Ward for their encouragement and advice; and Sisters Trina McGrath and Shanee Spencer, who have been sounding boards for my ideas. The staff of St Paul's and St Barbara's Wards and the Domiciliary Service of St Vincent's Hospital, Melbourne are gratefully acknowledged for enthusiastically participating in the evaluation of the draft Manual and providing valuable feedback about content, clarity and usefulness. I extend thanks to the nursing and medical administrative bodies of St Vincent's Hospital for permission to evaluate The Manual in the clinical setting.

Many thanks also to Dr Gordon Ennis, Professor Pincus Taft, Mary Rankin, Dr Beverley Wood, Marion Duff, Mrs Roberta Pearce and Anne Cook, who all read the manuscript and gave constructive comment about their specialist areas.

I am indebted to the library staff of St Vincent's Hospital, Sandra, Kathleen and Lorraine, who helped me track down resource material, found lost references and asked after progress.

To Nicole Hayes, who typed the first draft of the manuscript, thank you; to Liz Carr, who typed the manuscript, advised about setting out the material, and who became a friend, I owe a debt of gratitude.

I am grateful to Mary MacKinnon, who helped me obtain information specific to the United Kingdom. I am indebted to Lisa Field and Teresa Heapy of Blackwell Scientific Publications for advice during the final preparation of the manuscript.

The support and understanding of my family has been invaluable. My especial thanks and love go to my husband, John, who has been 'the wind beneath my wings'.

List of Abbreviations and Symbols

Listed alphabetically

↑	Increased
↓	Decreased
<	Less than
≥	Equal to, or greater than
>	Greater than
BG	Blood glucose
BP	Blood pressure
BUN	Blood urea nitrogen
CAPD	Continuous ambulatory peritoneal dialysis
CCF	Congestive cardiac failure
CCU	Coronary care unit
CSII	Continuous Subcutaneous insulin infusion
DA	Diabetes Australia
DKA	Diabetic ketoacidosis
ECG	Electrocardiogram
EN	Enteral nutrition
HbA1c	Glycosylated haemoglobin
HM	Human insulin
HONK	Hyperosmolar non-ketotic coma
ICU	Intensive care unit
IDDM	Insulin-dependent diabetes
IV	Intravenous therapy lines
LFT	Liver function test
NDSS	National Diabetes Supply Scheme
NIDDM	Non-insulin-dependent diabetes
OGTT	Oral glucose tolerance test
OHA	Oral hypoglycaemic agent
TPN	Total parenteral nutrition
TPR	Temperature, pulse and respiration

The words are used in full the first time they appear in the text. The abbreviations are listed here to assist those who read chapters at random. All abbreviations are widely accepted and recognized.

Chapter 1
Introduction

1.1 What is diabetes mellitus?

Diabetes mellitus is a metabolic disorder in which the body's capacity to utilize sugar, fat and protein is disturbed due to insulin deficiency or insulin resistance. Both states lead to an elevated blood glucose concentration and glycosuria.

The body is unable to utilize glucose in the absence of insulin and draws on fats and proteins in an effort to supply fuel for energy. Carbohydrate is necessary for the complete metabolism of fats, however, and when carbohydrate metabolism is disordered fat metabolism is incomplete and intermediate products (ketone bodies) can accumulate in the blood leading to ketosis, especially in Type 1 diabetes. The protein breakdown in this situation leads to weight loss and weakness and contributes to the development of hyperglycaemia and lethargy.

There are different types of diabetes which have different underlying causal mechanisms and clinical presentation. In general, young people are insulin-deficient (Type 1 diabetes), while older people may have sufficient insulin secretion and plasma insulin levels but demonstrate resistance to its action (Type 2 diabetes). Type 2 diabetes is the most common, accounting for 85% of diagnosed cases; Type 1 accounts for 15% of diagnosed cases.

1.2 Classification of diabetes

Diabetes can be loosely classified into:

- Type 1 or insulin-dependent diabetes (IDDM).
- Type 2 or non-insulin-dependent diabetes (NIDDM).
- Secondary diabetes.
- Gestational diabetes.
- Malnutrition-related diabetes (tropical diabetes).
- Maturity onset diabetes of the young (MODY).

Diabetes affects approximately 0.5 to 4% of the population depending on the type of diabetes, age group and ethnic group. The incidence of diabetes appears to be increasing, particularly in the older age group.

1.3   Presentation of Type 1 and Type 2 diabetes

1.3.1   Type 1 diabetes

Type 1 diabetes usually affects children and young adults. It often presents with the so-called classic symptoms of diabetes mellitus:

- Polyuria
- Polydipsia
- Lethargy
- Weight loss

These symptoms usually occur over a short space of time (two to three weeks) as a result of destruction of the beta cells of the pancreas. The precipitating event may have occurred many years prior to the development of the symptoms. Type 1 diabetes is an autoimmune disease. Blood glucose will be elevated and urinary glucose and ketones will be detected on testing. In severe cases the patient will present with diabetic ketoacidosis (DKA) (see Chapter 9).

1.3.2   Type 2 diabetes

Type 2 diabetes may present with an established long-term complication of diabetes such as neuropathy, cardiovascular disease or retinopathy. Alternatively, diabetes may be diagnosed during another illness or on routine screening. The classic symptoms described above are often less obvious and occur over a longer period of time. Once treatment is instituted people often recognize that they have more energy and are less thirsty.

People most at risk of developing Type 2 diabetes are:

- Overweight.
- Over 40 years of age.
- Closely related to people with diabetes.
- Women who have had gestational diabetes or who had large babies.

The characteristics of Type 1 and Type 2 diabetes are shown in Table 1.1.

1.3.3   Secondary diabetes

In some cases, diabetes occurs as a result of another disorder, for example pancreatic disease or endocrine disorders such as acromegaly and

Table 1.1   Characteristics of Type 1 and Type 2 diabetes mellitus.

	Type 1 Insulin-dependent (IDDM)	*Type 2 non-insulin-dependent (NIDDM)*
Age at onset	Usually < 30 years	Usually > 40 years
Body weight	Normal or underweight; often recent weight loss	80% are overweight
Heredity	Associated with specific human leukocyte antigen (HLA)	No HLA association
	Autoimmune disease	
	Viral infection possible trigger	No evidence for viral trigger
Insulin	Early insulin secretion Impaired later; may be totally absent	Insulin deficiency or resistance to insulin action
Ketosis	Common	Rare
Frequency	15% of diagnosed cases	85% of diagnosed cases
Complications	Common	Common

Cushing's disease. This is called secondary diabetes, which can also be precipitated by drugs such as cortisone and thiazide diuretics.

1.3.4   Gestational diabetes

Gestational diabetes is defined as carbohydrate intolerance of variable severity which is first recognized during pregnancy. It affects about 3% of all pregnant women. The exact cause of gestational diabetes is unknown, but several factors have been identified including insulin resistance and hyperglycaemia as a result of the hormones produced by the placenta.

Usually the blood glucose returns to normal after delivery of the baby. However, approximately 40% of women with gestational diabetes will develop diabetes in later life.

It is recommended that all pregnant women be screened for diabetes between 24 and 28 weeks gestation, the time the placenta begins to produce large quantities of hormones.

Who is At Risk from Gestational Diabetes?
Gestational diabetes can occur in any pregnancy, however those women at highest risk may be categorized as:

- Older.
- Overweight.
- Having a family history of diabetes or previous gestational diabetes or having had a large baby previously.
- Belonging to a race with an increased risk, e.g. Vietnamese.

If the blood glucose cannot be controlled by diet, insulin will usually be required during pregnancy. Oral hypoglycaemic agents (OHAs) are contraindicated because they cross the placenta and cause neonatal hypoglycaemia. The aim of treatment is to keep blood glucose within the normal range (3–7 mmol), ensure the diet is appropriate and provide good obstetric care.

1.3.5   Malnutrition-related (tropical) diabetes

Childhood malnutrition, genetic predisposition and environmental factors are implicated in the development of diabetes in people living in tropical countries. 'Tropical diabetes' or malnutrition-related diabetes differs from Type 1 diabetes because ketoacidosis is rare, and from Type 2 diabetes because it often occurs in young, thin people with no family history of diabetes. However, researchers have not yet agreed about the underlying causal mechanisms.

1.3.6   Maturity onset diabetes of the young (MODY)

Maturity onset diabetes of the young is a rare subgroup of Type 2 diabetes, also called Mason-type diabetes and non-insulin-dependent diabetes of the young (NIDDY). It usually occurs in young people less than 25 years of age. It was originally thought to be an autosomal dominant inheritance, but considerable genetic heterogenicity has been described between different races. MODY can be distinguished from Type 1 diabetes by the absence of ketosis. Treatment is with oral hypoglycaemic agents, diet and exercise, although insulin may eventually be required.

1.4   Diagnosis of diabetes

Urine tests alone should not be used to make a diagnosis of diabetes; if glycosuria is detected the blood glucose should be tested. When symptoms of diabetes are present an elevated blood glucose alone will usually confirm the diagnosis (fasting >7.8 mmol/l; random >11 mmol/l).

If the person is asymptomatic, abnormal fasting blood glucose values (>8 mmol/l) should be demonstrated on at least two occasions before the diagnosis is made. A random plasma glucose of >11 mmol/l two hours after a meal is diagnostic of diabetes. An oral glucose tolerance test (OGTT) using a 75 g glucose load may be indicated to determine the presence of glucose intolerance if results are borderline. The criteria for diagnosing diabetes according to the World Health Organization are shown in Table 1.2. For performance of test and patient preparation for an OGTT see section 1.5.

Table 1.2   Diagnostic criteria for the diagnosis of diabetes following a 75 g oral glucose tolerance test.

| | Venous plasma glucose level (mmol/l) | |
	Fasting	2 hours after food
Normal glucose tolerance	<6.0	<8.0
Impaired glucose tolerance test	<7.8	7.8–11
Diabetes mellitus	>7.8	>11.1

In this table venous plasma glucose values are shown. Glucose in capillary blood is about 10–15% higher than venous blood.

1.5   Oral glucose tolerance test (OGTT)

An OGTT is used only:

● When fasting and random blood glucose results are equivocal.
● When there is a strong family history of diabetes, especially during pregnancy.
● If the suspicion of diabetes is high but blood and urine glucose tests are normal.

An OGTT should not be performed when the patient:

● Is febrile.
● Is acutely ill (e.g. post-operatively, or if uraemic).
● Has been immobilized for more than 48 hours.
● Has symptoms of diabetes or elevated blood glucose before commencement of the test.

1.5.1   Preparation of the patient for an OGTT

(1) Give adequate oral and written instructions to the patient. A sample is given in Patient Instruction Sheet 1.

(2) Ensure the diet contains at least 200 g/day carbohydrate 3 to 5 days pretest.

(3) If possible stop drugs which may influence the test 3 days before the test:
- thiazide diuretics
- antihypertensive drugs
- analgesic and anti-inflammatory drugs
- anti-neoplastic drugs
- steroids.

(4) Fast from 12 midnight before the test.

(5) Avoid physical/psychological stress for 1 hour prior to, and during, the test.

(6) Avoid smoking for at least 1 hour prior to the test.

(7) Allow the patient to relax 30 minutes before beginning the test.

1.5.2   Test protocol

(1) A cannula is inserted into a suitable vein for blood sampling.

(2) The blood glucose should be tested before commencing the test. If elevated clarify with the doctor ordering the test before proceeding. Two ml of blood are collected in fluoride oxalate tubes for laboratory analysis.

(3) The cannula is flushed with saline or heparinized saline between samples to prevent clotting.

(4) Blood samples are collected at:

minutes:		
	−10	
	0	
	⇨	75 g glucose, consumed over 5 minutes
	+ 30	
	+ 60	
	+ 120	

The glucose is prepacked in 300 ml bottles containing exactly 75 g of glucose (usually available from hospital pharmacies).

1.6   Management of diabetes mellitus

1.6.1   The diabetes team

Diabetes management is considered to be team care. The patient is a key player in the team. Good communication between team members is

PATIENT INSTRUCTION SHEET 1: PREPARATION FOR AN ORAL GLUCOSE TOLERANCE TEST

PATIENT INSTRUCTIONS FOR ORAL GLUCOSE TOLERANCE TEST

Date of test: Name:

Time: UR:

Location where test will take place:

---

(1) Please ensure that you eat high carbohydrate meals each day for 3 days before the test. Carbohydrate foods are: breads, cereals, spaghetti, noodles, rice, dried beans and pulses, vegetables, fruit. These foods should constitute the major part of your diet for the 3 days.

(2) Have nothing to eat or drink after 12 midnight on the night prior to the test day, except water.

(3) Bring a list of all the tablets you are taking with you when you come for the test.

(4) Do not smoke for at least one hour before the test.

The Test

The test is performed in the morning. You are required to rest during the test, which will take approximately 3 hours to complete. A small needle will be inserted into an arm vein for blood sampling. The needle will stay in place until the test is completed. You will be given 300 ml of glucose to drink. This is very sweet but it is important to drink it all over the 5 minutes, so that the results of the test can be interpreted correctly.

You will be given a cup of tea and something to eat when the test is finished. The doctor will discuss the results with you.

important and information given to the patient must be consistent between, and within, departments. The team usually consists of some or all of the following:

- Diabetologist
- Diabetes educator
- Dietitian
- Podiatrist
- Social worker
- Psychologist
- General practitioner

Other professionals who contribute regularly to the management of the patient are:

- Opthalmologist
- Renal physician
- Pharmacist
- Vascular and orthopaedic surgeons

The ward staff who care for the patient in hospital also become team members:

- Nurses
- Physiotherapists
- Occupational therapists

The management of diabetes is based on dietary modification, regular exercise/activity and in some cases insulin or OHAs. Diabetes education and regular medical assessment of diabetic control and complication status is essential.

1.6.2   Aim of management

The aim of diabetes management is to keep the patient free from the symptoms of diabetes, and the blood glucose in an acceptable range. The range is determined on an individual basis, usually between 4 and 10 mmol/l for 90% of tests. However in young people and during pregnancy the aim is to obtain results as near as possible to normal blood glucose levels (fasting 4–8 mmol/l and <10 mmol/l after food). To achieve this, there must be a balance between the food plan, medication (insulin/OHAs) and exercise/activity. The regime should restrict lifestyle as little as possible, although some modification is usually necessary. Type 1 (insulin-dependent) people require insulin in order to survive. Type 2 (non-insulin-dependent) obese patients can be treated effectively with a combination of diet and exercise. In many people with Type 2 diabetes OHAs will also be required, and sometimes eventually insulin.

Table 1.3 Guidelines for assessment of control of diabetes.

% haemoglobin A1c	Glucose (mmol/l)		Control
	Fasting	2 hours after food	
4.0–6.0	4	7.0	Excellent or 'too good'
6.0–7.4	7.0	10	Very good or excellent
7.5–9.4	10	14.5	Acceptable but fair only
>9.5	14	20	Poor

Management involves education of the person with diabetes and other family members in order to:

- Obtain and maintain an acceptable weight.
- Achieve acceptable blood glucose levels.
- Achieve a normal blood lipid profile.
- Relieve symptoms of diabetes (polyuria, polydipsia and lethargy).
- Prevent complications of diabetes and of treatment.
- Maintain a healthy independent lifestyle where the person is able to manage the necessary self-care tasks to achieve acceptable glycaemic control.

Some guidelines for assessing diabetic control are shown in Table 1.3.

1.6.3 Exercise/activity

Exercise plays a key role in the management of both Type 1 and Type 2 diabetes. It increases tissue sensitivity to insulin aiding in the uptake and utilization of glucose during exercise and for several hours afterwards. The energy sources during exercise are depicted in Fig. 1.1.

In addition regular exercise:

- Increases cardiovascular efficiency.
- Decreases blood pressure.
- Reduces stress.
- Aids in weight reduction and appetite control.
- Promotes a sense of well-being.
- Aids in blood glucose control.

All of these factors also decrease the risk of developing the long-term complications of diabetes. People are advised to have a thorough physical check-up before commencing an exercise programme; in particular, the cardiovascular system, eyes, nerves and feet should be examined. The

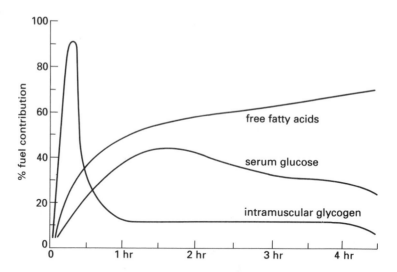

Fig. 1.1   Normal energy sources during exercise.

Note: At rest free fatty acids are the major energy source. As exercise begins muscle
glycogen is utilized as the predominant energy source. As exercise continues the
blood glucose is utilized, reverting to free fatty acids as the major energy source if
exercise is prolonged. Blood glucose is maintained by hormonal regulation of hepatic
glucose output and lipolysis.

exercise chosen should be suited to the person's physical condition. It is
advisable to test the blood glucose before and after exercising and to have
some carbohydrate available during exercise in case of hypoglycaemia.
Infrequent exercise is not advisable; the aim should be to exercise three to
five times per week for 30 to 40 minutes each time. Footwear should be
appropriate to the type of exercise and the feet inspected after exercising.
Exercise is not recommended in extremes of temperatures, or at periods of
poor diabetic control, especially if ketones are present in the urine. People
should discuss their exercise plans with the diabetes team in order to plan
an appropriate routine, adequate carbohydrate intake, and appropriate
medication dose.

Hypoglycaemia can occur hours after the exercise is completed and extra
carbohydrate may be needed.

In general, anaerobic exercise (e.g. weight lifting) does not use glucose as
a fuel. This type of exercise builds muscle mass, but does not improve the
cardiovascular system. Anaerobic exercise is likely to cause an increase in
blood glucose. Aerobic exercise (running, cycling, swimming) uses glucose
as the major fuel source and a decrease in blood glucose can occur. It also
confers cardiovascular benefits.

1.6.4 Exercise for the patient in hospital

(1) Encourage as much mobility/activity as the patient's condition allows.
(2) Ambulate gradually after a period of being confined to bed.
(3) Consult the physiotherapy department for assistance with mobility, chair or hydrotherapy exercises.

Be aware that the first time out of bed after prolonged inactivity constitutes unaccustomed exercise and can result in hypoglycaemia.

1.7 Diabetes education

Diabetes education is an important part of diabetes management. Regular support and contact with the diabetes care team assists people to manage their diabetes by providing advice and support when necessary. For more details see Chapter 18.

Type 2 patients *do not* become Type 1 when insulin is needed to control blood glucose levels. They are termed 'insulin-requiring' diabetics. Insulin is needed to control the blood glucose but usually some endogenous insulin production still occurs. Except in severe intercurrent illnesses, ketoacidosis is prevented by this insulin production.

1.8 Complications of diabetes

Many admissions of people with diabetes to hospital are a result of one or more of the complications of diabetes. The presence of a diabetic complication can affect the duration of the admission and the patient's ability to care for him/herself. Hence diabetic complications contribute to the overall cost of health care for these patients.

Complications can be classified as acute or long-term. Acute complications can occur if diabetic management is not optimal; long-term complications are thought to be partially a result of chronic hyperglycaemia (poor control). Often more than one complication is co-existent in the one patient.

1.8.1 Acute complications

(1) Hypoglycaemia (refer to Chapter 8).
(2) Hyperglycaemia:
   - diabetic ketoacidosis (refer to Chapter 10)
   - hyperosmolar coma (refer to Chapter 10).

(3) Infections can occur if blood glucose control is not optimal. Common infections include candidiasis and urinary tract infections.

(4) Fat atrophy/hypertrophy and insulin allergy occur very rarely with modern highly purified insulins and correct site rotation.

1.8.2 Chronic complications

(1) Macrovascular disease or disease of the major blood vessels, e.g.:
  ● myocardial infarction
  ● cerebrovascular accident
  ● intermittent claudication.

(2) Microvascular disease or disease of the small blood vessels associated with thickening of the basement membranes of the vessels, e.g.:
  ● retinopathy
  ● nephropathy.

(3) Neuropathy: diabetes can also cause damage to the central and peripheral nerves:
  ● peripheral: decreased sensation in hands and feet, which can lead to foot ulcers
  ● autonomic: impotence, atonic bladder, gastric paresis, mono-neuropathies.

(4) Complications of pregnancy: diabetes during pregnancy carries risks for both mother and baby:
  ● mother: toxaemia, polyhydramnous intrauterine death, caesarian section
  ● baby: congenital malformations, prematurity, respiratory distress, hypoglycaemia at birth.

It is not the purpose of this Manual to discuss the mechanisms and pathophysiology behind the development of diabetic complications. A list of recommended reading which deals with this subject has been included in Appendix B

It is the responsibility of the nurse to assess the patient adequately for the presence of complications in order to devise an appropriate nursing care plan, and to be involved in preventative teaching about reducing risk factors for the development of diabetic complications.

1.9 Cost of diabetes

The Australian Institute of Health in 1991 estimated the cost of diabetes in Australia to be $7000 million per year. The cost of diabetes in the UK was estimated at £1 billion, according to National Health Services figures of 1989. These costs are increasing, especially for older people. In addition, the length of stay in hospital is longer for people with diabetes. Many of the hospitalizations are a result of diabetic complications which should be largely preventable.

Sixty per cent of the costs associated with diabetes are direct costs of providing service and medical supplies. The indirect costs (40%) are more difficult to assess; they include psychological costs to the person with diabetes, life years lost and loss of quality of life. There are also costs to the care-givers (relatives and family) which cannot be estimated.

Diabetes is the fourth major cause of death after cardiovascular disease, cancer and musculo-skeletal disease, distributed across all age groups. Cardiovascular disease is a major complication of diabetes. Therefore it is not unreasonable to conclude that a person with diabetes will require at least one hospital contact/admission during their lifetime. It is documented that the need for hospital admission and the length of stay in hospital can be improved by diabetes education, and appropriate medical and nursing care. It is envisaged that this Manual will contribute to the provision of that care.

1.10   Aim and objectives of nursing care of people with diabetes

1.10.1   Aim

To formulate an individual nursing management plan so that the patient recovers by primary intention, maintains independence as far as possible and does not develop any complications of treatment.

1.10.2   Objectives

(1) To assess the patient's:
  - physical, mental and social status
  - usual diabetic control
  - ability to care for themselves
  - knowledge about diabetes and its management
  - the presence of any diabetes-related complications
  - acceptance of the diagnosis of diabetes.
(2) To encourage independence as far as the physical condition allows in hospital (test own blood glucose, administer own insulin, select own meals).
(3) To obtain and maintain an acceptable blood glucose range, thereby preventing hypoglycaemia or hyperglycaemia so that the patient is free from distressing symptoms of fluctuating blood glucose levels.

(4) To prevent complications occurring as a result of hospitalization (e.g. falls).

(5) To observe an appropriate nursing care plan in order to achieve these objectives.

(6) To inform appropriate health professionals (e.g. diabetes educator, dietitian, podiatrist) of the patient's admission.

(7) To ensure patient has the opportunity to learn about diabetes and its management, particularly self-management.

(8) To plan appropriately for discharge.

(9) To prevent further hospitalizations as a result of diabetes.

Chapter 2
Patient Assessment/Nursing Diagnosis

2.1 Key points

- Assess general nursing needs.
- Incorporate diabetic assessment.
- Formulate individual care plans.
- Begin with the nursing history.
- Evaluate treatment outcomes.
- Discharge planning should be part of the care plan.

2.2 Characteristics of the nursing history

The nursing history:

- Begins with demographic data (age, sex, social situation).
- Collects units of information to permit individual care plans.
- Obtains baseline information.
- Should be concise to allow information to be collected in a short time.
- Allows formulation of an individual nursing care plan taking into account the patient's expectations of the care.
- Assists in maintaining independence while in hospital (e.g. allowing patient to perform own blood glucose tests).

The findings should be documented in the patient record and communicated to the appropriate caregivers.

Note: A guideline for obtaining a comprehensive nursing history follows. It is important however to listen to the patient and not be locked into 'ticking boxes', so that vital and valuable information is not overlooked.

Most of the information is general in nature, but some will be specifically relevant to diabetes (e.g. blood glucose testing and eating patterns). The clinical assessment in this example is particularly aimed at obtaining information about diabetic status.

Assessment of the person with diabetes does not differ from the assessment performed for any other disease process. Assessment should take into account social, physical and psychological factors in order to prepare an appropriate nursing care plan including a plan for discharge.

Any physical disability the patient has will affect his/her ability to self-manage their diabetes (inject insulin, inspect feet, test blood glucose). Impaired hearing may preclude group education programmes. Management and educational expectations may need to be modified to take any disability into account.

The diagnosis of diabetes, however, means that metabolic derangements may be present at admission, or could develop as a consequence of hospitalization. Therefore careful assessment allows for a co-ordinated nursing care plan and appropriate referral to other health professionals (podiatrist, diabetes educator, dietitian). A nursing problem list, ranking problems in order of priority, can also assist in planning individualized care to address immediate and future treatment goals. The first step in patient assessment is to document a nursing history.

2.3 Nursing History

A nursing history is a written record of specific information about a patient. The data collected allows the nurse to plan appropriate nursing actions and to incorporate patient needs. A good patient care plan will allow consistency of treatment expectations within, and between, departments. An example patient assessment chart is shown in Patient Care Sheet 1.

PATIENT CARE SHEET 1:
EXAMPLE OF A PATIENT ASSESSMENT CHART,
FORMULATED FOR PEOPLE WITH DIABETES

EXAMPLE OF A PATIENT ASSESSMENT CHART

Formulated for People with Diabetes

A.   GUIDELINES FOR OBTAINING A NURSING HISTORY

Name: ....

Age: ....   Sex: ☐ Male ☐ Female

Type of diabetes: ☐ IDDM ☐ NIDDM ☐ Other

Social

Language spoken: ....

Command of English: ☐ Written ☐ Spoken

Marital status: ....

Living arrangements: ☐ With partner ☐ Alone

Support systems: ....

Work type: ....

Meals

Regular meals: ☐ Yes ☐ No

Who does the cooking: ....

Eating out: ....

Alcohol consumption: ☐ Yes ☐ No   How much: ....

How often: ....

PATIENT CARE SHEET 1 *contd*

Smoking

☐ Yes ☐ No   Cigarettes/pipe: ....

How many per day: ....   Marijuana: ....

Current Medications

General: ....

Diabetic: ....

Usual Activity Level

Sports: ....

Gardening: ....

Walking: ....

Other: ....

Disabilities

What activities are limited: ....

To what degree: ....

(1)   General: ....

(2)   Hearing: ....

(3)   Related to diabetic complications:

       Decreased vision: ....

       Neuropathy: (a) Peripheral: ....

                      (b) Autonomic: ....

       Vascular: (a) Cardiac: ....

                      (b) Legs and feet: ....

       Kidney function: ....

       Sexuality: (a) Impotence: ....

(4)   Mobility: ....

(5)   Dexterity (fine motor skills): ....

PATIENT CARE SHEET 1 *contd*

Self-Monitoring of Diabetic Control (Testing Methods)

Urine test: ☐ Glucose ☐ Ketones   Strips used: ....

Tests own blood glucose: ☐ Yes ☐ No

Testing frequency: ....

System used:

(1)   Visual, BM strips, glucostix, betacheck: ....

(2)   Blood Glucose Meter Type: ....

Testing accuracy: ....

Insulin technique/accuracy: ....

Drawing up: ....

Administration: ....

Type of insulin: ....

Patient can name type of insulin: ☐ Yes ☐ No

Frequency of dose: ....

Psychological Adjustment to Diabetes

☐ Anxiety ☐ Denial ☐ Depression ☐ Well adjusted

Mental state: ....

Diabetic Knowledge Assessment

Previous diabetes education: ☐ Yes ☐ No

Attendance at education support groups: ☐ Yes ☐ No

Name of group: ....

How assessed: ....

PATIENT CARE SHEET 1 *contd*

Patient's Stated Reason for Being In Hospital

....

....

B.   CLINICAL EXAMINATION

A detailed physical examination of the patient is carried out by the medical staff, however there is also a place for clinical examination of the patient by the nursing staff. Particular attention should be paid to the following areas.

(1)   General Inspection

- Conscious state
- temperature, pulse and respiration
- blood pressure lying and standing; note any postural drop
- height
- weight and history of weight gain/loss
- hydration status, skin turgor
- presence of diabetic symptoms, thirst, polyuria, polydipsia, lethargy
- full urinalysis
- blood glucose.

PATIENT CARE SHEET 1 *contd*

(2)   Skin

- Pigmentation
- skin tone/turgor, colour
- presence of lesions, rashes, wounds, ulcers
- inspect injection sites, including abdomen; note any thickening, lumps, bruises.

(3)   Mouth

- Mucous membranes, (dry/moist)
- lips
- infection, halitosis
- teeth: evidence of dental caries, loose teeth, red gums, incorrectly fitting dentures.

(4)   Feet and Legs

- The skin of the feet and legs may be hairless and shiny due to poor circulation
- muscle wasting
- ulcers or pressure areas on soles of feet and toes, including old scars
- loss of pain sensation which may be due to nerve damage; estimate the size and depth of ulcers
- presence of oedema
- infection including fungal infection; inspect between the toes
- condition of nails and general cleanliness of feet.

Chapter 3
Documenting and Charting Patient Care

3.1 Documenting in the medical record

3.1.1 Nursing care plans

The employing institution's policy regarding the method of documentation should be followed. Good nursing documentation allows communication of the care required, to all staff. In the future changes will occur to the methods of documenting care; for example narrative notes may be replaced by focus charting and flow charts. Flow charts are designed to enable all health care providers to document care on a single care plan. Much of the current duplication can thus be avoided.

Standardized care plans of common medical and nursing diagnosis are being developed to serve as blueprints and may reduce the time spent on documentation. In the future many of the data may be entered on computers at the patient's bedside as is already occurring in the USA. When standard care plans are used it is vital to assess and document individual patient needs. Figure 3.1 is an example of a patient care flow chart to illustrate the use of standard patient care plans.

3.1.2 Nursing notes

The progress notes are a record of the patient's hospital admission and response to treatment, and act as a guide for discharge planning. They should be written legibly and objectively. They are not legal documents but may be subpoenaed for a court hearing.

Document the following:

- The condition of the patient objectively; for example, describe wounds in terms of size and depth.
- Qualification of the patient's condition, recording swelling, oedema, temperature, pulse and respiration (TPR) and blood pressure (BP).
- All teaching the patient receives.
- The patient's response to treatment.
- All medications received.
- Removal of all invasive medical devices (e.g. packs, drains, IV lines).

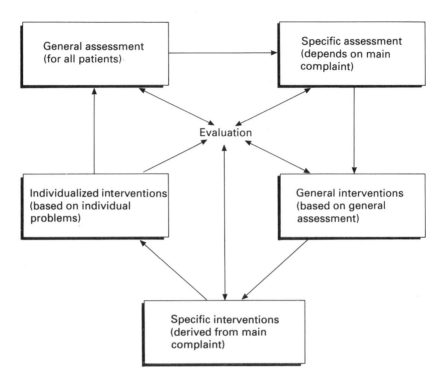

Fig. 3.1   Flow chart to illustrate the use of standard patient care plans. (Based on Fig. 3.5 in Walsh, M. (1990) *Accident and Emergency Nursing.* Heinemann Nursing, Oxford. Reproduced with permission.)

3.1.3 Diabetic chart

The purpose of the chart is:

- To provide a record of blood and urinary glucose measurements.
- To record ketones in urine.
- To provide a record of the amount and time of administration of insulin/ oral hypoglycaemic agent doses.
- To record episodes of hypoglycaemia.
- To provide a basis for the adjustment of insulin/oral hypoglycaemic agents.

Frequency of blood and urine testing is dependent on the patient's status and the treatment being given (*see* Chapter 4).

DIABETIC FREQUENT MONITORING

IDENTIFICATION

DATE	TIME	INSULIN		BLOOD SUGAR	URINE							ACETONE	PROTEIN	NURSING COMMENTS E.g. Adverse reactions or food omission
		TYPE	DOSE		GLUCOSE									
					0 %	1/10 %	1/4 %	1/2 %	1 %	2 %				

(a)

INSTRUCTIONS
TYPE OF INSULIN, BLOOD GLUCOSE AND
URINE TESTS MUST BE RECORDED IN FULL.

IDENTIFICATION

Date		0700	1100	1600	2100	COMMENTS
	Insulin type					
	Dose					
	Blood glucose mmols/l					
	Urine glucose					
	Ketones					
	Insulin type					
	Dose					
	Blood glucose mmols/l					
	Urine glucose					
	Ketones					

(b)

Fig. 3.2   Sample diabetic record charts for (a) 2 hourly testing (e.g. when using an insulin infusion); (b) 4 hourly or less frequent testing.

3.2 Nursing responsibilities

(1) Write legibly.
(2) Record all medication doses accurately in the correct column.
(3) Record hypoglycaemic episodes (symptoms, treatment, time, activity and food omission) in the appropriate column. Hypoglycaemia should also be documented in the patient's unit record.
(4) Do not add unnecessary details.

Figure 3.2 depicts example charts for (a) frequent testing and (b) testing 4 hourly or less often.

Chapter 4
Monitoring Diabetes Mellitus

4.1 Introduction

Monitoring of blood and urine glucose is an important part of diabetes management. The results obtained form the basis for adjusting medication, food intake and activity levels. Urine glucose is no longer the major method of assessing metabolic control, but is still useful for some people, provided the renal threshold for glucose has been established.

Patients are expected to monitor their diabetes at home. They should be encouraged to continue to self-monitor in hospital if they are well enough to do so. Always inform the patient of the result of the blood or urine glucose test. This time can be used as teaching time.

The results of blood and urine tests are only useful if tests are accurately performed.

Monitoring 1: blood glucose

4.2 Key points

- Get a good drop of blood.
- Time accurately.
- Remove blood correctly.
- Calibrate and clean meter regularly.
- Record and interpret results.

4.3 The role of blood glucose monitoring in the care of diabetes

Blood glucose monitoring provides insight into the effectiveness of the diabetes management plan. It allows the patient direct feedback about factors which influence blood glucose.

Blood glucose testing is performed to:

- Monitor the effectiveness of diabetes therapy: food plan, OHAs/insulin, exercise/activity.
- Detect lack of control as indicated by elevated glycosylated haemoglobin (HbA1c) levels.
- Achieve better control and acceptable blood glucose levels which may have a role in preventing or delaying the onset of diabetes-related complications.
- Diagnose hypoglycaemia including nocturnal hypoglycaemia, which may present as sleep disturbances.
- Establish the renal threshold and therefore the reliability of urine testing.
- Achieve 'tight' control in pregnancy and thereby reduce the risks to both mother and baby.
- Provide continuity of care following hospitalization.

Blood glucose monitoring is of particular use in:

- Frequent hypoglycaemic episodes.
- Unstable or 'brittle' diabetes.
- Management of illnesses at home, and in those recovering from an illness.
- Pregnancy.
- Establishing a new treatment regime.
- Patients with unreliable urine tests.
- Outpatient stabilization onto insulin.
- Patients with renal failure, autonomic neuropathy, cardiovascular or

cerebrovascular insufficiency where hypoglycaemic signs may be masked or not recognized.

The target blood glucose range and frequency of testing should be assessed individually.

4.3.1 Factors which influence blood glucose levels

(1) Food: times of last food intake, quantity and type of carbohydrate/ fibre consumed.
(2) Exercise: timing with respect to food, medication and insulin injection site.
(3) Intercurrent illness, e.g. influenza, urinary tract infection.
(4) Medications used for diabetes control: oral agents, insulin.
(5) Other drugs, e.g. steroids, oral contraceptives, beta blockers.
(6) Alcohol: type, relationship to food intake, amount consumed.
(7) Insulin type, injection site, injection technique.
(8) Emotional and physical stress – not only stress itself but medications used to treat stress.
(9) Accuracy of monitoring technique, including not handwashing before testing if sweet substances have been handled.
(10) Pregnancy in people with diabetes and gestational diabetes.
(11) Childhood: erratic swings in blood glucose levels are common.
(12) Adolescence: hormonal factors during adolescence make control difficult.
(13) Renal, liver and pancreatic disease.
(14) Other endocrine disorders, eg. thyroid disease, Cushing's disease.
(15) Patients on parenteral nutrition.

Insulin absorption can be delayed if injected into an oedemateous or ascitic abdomen. The upper arm may be a preferable site in this instance.

4.4 Guidelines for the frequency of blood glucose monitoring

(1) Capillary blood glucose tests should be performed only by adequately qualified nursing and medical staff.
(2) Medical staff are responsible for interpreting the results and adjusting diabetes treatment accordingly.

These are guidelines only; refer to the policy and procedure manual of the employing institution.

4.4.1 Suggested protocol

Blood glucose and urinalysis are performed before meals and before bed (standard times are 7 AM, 11 AM, 4 PM and 9 PM), in order to obtain a profile of the effectiveness of diabetes therapy and to establish the renal threshold. Tests may also be performed 2 hours after food to provide information about glucose clearance from the blood stream. Results should usually be <10 mmol/l. Tests may be performed at 2 AM or 3 AM for two to three days to ascertain if nocturnal hypoglycaemia is occurring.

Urine ketones should be monitored in all patients with insulin-dependent diabetes and in some non-insulin-dependent people during severe stress (e.g. surgery, infection, myocardial infarctions, etc.) if blood glucose tests are elevated. Each patient should be assessed individually and the testing schedule tailored to individual requirements.

4.4.2 Regime for patients on insulin

Initially, for 48 hours, monitor at 7 AM, 11 AM, 4 PM and 9 PM to assess the effectiveness of current insulin therapy. Review and alter if indicated. If the insulin regimen is altered, continue tests as above and review again in 48 hours.

4.4.3 Patients on oral hypoglycaemic agents

Initial monitoring as for insulin controlled patients. Review at 48 hours as above. Decrease monitoring to twice daily, daily or once every second or third day, alternating the times of testing, as indicated by the level of control and the general medical condition of the patient.

4.4.4 Patients controlled by diet

Initially, twice daily monitoring, decreasing to daily or once every second or third day, unless the patient is undergoing surgery or actually ill.

4.4.5 Special circumstances

These will require individual orders by medical staff. They include:

(1) Insulin infusion: tests are usually performed every 2 hours during the infusion and reviewed every 2 hours. Reduce to 3 to 4 hourly when stable.
(2) Steroid therapy
  (a) non-diabetic patients: alternate weeks only, unless results are abnormal;

(b) diabetic: see protocols in sections 4.4.2, 4.4.3 or 4.4.4.
(3) Total parenteral nutrition (TPN) guidelines suggest:
  (a) routine blood glucose testing for the first 48 hours, 7 AM, 11 AM, 4 PM and 9 PM, until the patient is stable on TPN, then revert to protocol in section 4.4.2 or 4.4.3;
  (b) routine urinalysis for glucose/ketones, 7 AM, 11 AM, 4 PM and 9 PM.

Never prick the feet except in babies, where heel pricks are preferred.

4.5   Blood glucose meters

Blood glucose meters are devices used to monitor blood glucose in the home or at the bedside in hospital. Technology of both meters and strips is changing rapidly. Staff should become familiar with the system in use in their place of employment. There are several meters in common use:

(1) Light reflectance meters
  ● Reflolux S, Accutrend (Boehringer Mannheim).
  ● Glucometer GX, Glucometer 3, Glucometer M+ (Bayer Diagnostics).
  ● Hypocount, Hypocount Supreme (General Diabetes Services).
(2) Electronic devices
  ● ExacTech Pen, Satellite G (Farmitalia Carla Erbo).

Meters must be cleaned and control tested regularly and calibrated appropriately according to the manufacturer's directions.

Blood glucose meters are *not* infallible. Incorrect operator technique is the major cause of inaccurate results.

4.6   Reasons for inaccurate blood glucose results

Inaccurate blood glucose readings can occur for the following reasons:

(1) Meters
  ● using the incorrect strip for the meter
  ● using the incorrect calibration or code
  ● inserting the strip incorrectly or facing the wrong way
  ● insufficient blood on the strip will give a false low reading
  ● using an unclean meter
  ● low or flat battery.

(2) Both meters and visual comparisons
- blood wiped from the strip too soon can give low readings
- blood left on the strip too long can give high readings
- incomplete removal of blood from the strip makes interpretation difficult
- touching the pad of the finger onto some test strips (BM strips) leads to patchy colour development and difficulty in interpreting colours
- strips used after expiry date may not be accurate
- failure to wash hands before testing, especially if sweet substances have been handled
- humidity and high temperatures affect some testing systems.

If in doubt repeat the test or confirm biochemically.

Meter and strip technology is changing rapidly. A 'no wipe' technology has been developed which limits the possibility of blood contamination during wiping/blotting. It is important to use the correct technique for each strip. Some no wipe strips have limited visual comparison.

Figure 4.1 outlines the steps to be taken when performing quality control testing of blood glucose monitoring equipment.

4.7 Further Reading

Package inserts supplied with all reagent strips.
Blood glucose meter operator instructions.

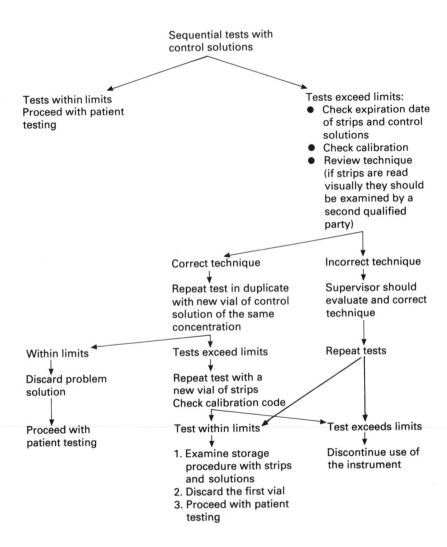

Fig. 4.1 Quality control flow chart for blood glucose testing.

PATIENT CARE SHEET 2:
BLOOD GLUCOSE TESTING CHECKLIST

BLOOD GLUCOSE TESTING CHECKLIST

Nursing Actions

(1)   Assemble materials and prepare environment according to hospital policy and testing system used.

- •   Remove test strip from vial and replace cap immediately
- •   dry cotton or rayon ball or tissue if required
- •   watch with a second hand depending on system used
- •   fingerpricking device (glucolet 2 preferred in hospital setting)
- •   well-lit environment.

(2)   Explain procedure to patient.

Obtaining a Drop of Blood

(1)   Wash patient's hands with soap and warm water, dry carefully.

(2)   Choose a site on any finger, near the side or tip. Avoid using the pad of the finger where nerves and arteries are concentrated; it is more painful.

(3)   Prick finger firmly, preferably using a fingerprick device.

(4)   Squeeze finger to well up blood at the puncture site, milking along the length of the finger.

(5)   Allow the drop of blood to fall onto the strip; do not rub onto the surface of strip.

Completing the Test

(1)   Use exact timing to allow glucose and reagent to react.

(2)   Remove all blood from strip at appropriate time depending on system used.

PATIENT CARE SHEET 2 *contd*

(3)   Wait the required time to allow full colour development. If appropriate obtain result in blood glucose meter, or in bright light visually compare colour on strip with colour blocks on strip container. BM 20/800 GLYCAEMIC STRIPS, GLUCOSTIX

(4)   Identify colour block whose colours are most like test strip's colours, and record blood glucose value assigned to that colour block.

(5)   Record test results on diabetes chart and in any other pertinent record.

(6)   Communicate results to appropriate person (doctor).

(7)   Dispose of sharps into appropriate sharps container.

Tips

(a)   Warm hands bleed more readily.

(b)   If peripheral circulation is deficient, obtaining blood can be difficult. Trap blood in fingertip with one hand, by milking the length of the finger and applying pressure with finger before pricking.

(c)   Prick finger.

(d)   Squeeze as above.

(e)   Ensure blood is applied to the centre of the reagent pad; check visually.

(f)   Insufficient blood will give a lower reading or an error message with most meters.

(g)   Check with biochemistry result.

Monitoring 2: urine glucose/ketones

4.8 Key points

- Establish renal threshold to determine reliability of urine tests.
- Hydration status affects results.
- Double voiding is unnecessary.
- Test for ketones if blood glucose is elevated, especially in Type 1 diabetics.
- Perform a full ward urine test on admission.

4.9 Introduction

In the presence of normal kidney function glycosuria is correlated to the blood glucose concentration. Glycosuria occurs when the tubular maximum reabsorption has been exceeded, usually around 8–10 mmol/l blood glucose. This is called the renal threshold for glucose and varies within and between individuals. The renal threshold may be changed by:

- Age
- Renal disease
- Long-standing diabetes

Therefore:

- The blood glucose can be elevated without glycosuria.
- Traces of glucose in the urine may indicate loss of control.
- The renal threshold may be low in children and glycosuria present when blood glucose is normal.

It is important to establish the renal threshold at a period of good control by simultaneously testing blood and urine glucose.

Urine glucose monitoring does not give warning of impending hypoglycaemia and a negative urine glucose finding does not indicate hypoglycaemia.

4.10 Limitations of urine glucose testing

(1) The degree of hydration influences the glucose concentration.
(2) The time since voiding influences the result.
(3) Urine glucose is a limited predictor of blood glucose.

4.11   Indications for urine glucose tests

(1) Type 2 diabetes.
(2) Very well controlled stable patients.
(3) When the aim is to avoid glycosuria.

Double voiding prior to testing is no longer considered necessary.

The currently available urine test strips are depicted in Table 4.1. Clinitest tablets are no longer the first choice method for urine testing, as they are more subject to interference by other compounds in the urine and to user error. They can cause chemical burns to the mouth if ingested. Moderate to heavy ketones in the urine can depress the colour reaction for glucose on Diastix and Ketodiastix. Blood glucose tests should be performed if ketones are present in the urine.

Table 4.1   Currently available urine test strips.

Trade name	Manufacturer	Uses
Clinistix Bottles of 100 strips	Ames–Bayer	Test for urine glucose
Diastix Bottles of 100 strips	Ames–Bayer	Test for urine glucose
Keto-diabur-Test 5000	Boehringer Mannheim	Test for both glucose and ketones
Ketodiastix Bottles of 100 strips	Ames–Bayer	Test for both glucose and ketones
Ketostix Bottles of 100 strips	Ames–Bayer	Test only for ketones

All urine test strips have a graded colour scale on the label to estimate the amount of glucose/ketones in the urine.

4.12   Monitoring of ketones

Ketone testing is important during illness in:

● All Type 1 diabetics.
● Type 2 people who are severely ill.

Ketonuria is a consequence of:

● Insulin deficiency.
● Starvation.
● Post-severe hypoglycaemia.
● Severe stress.

4.13   Urine tests of kidney function

Twelve and 24 hour collections of urine are used to monitor kidney function and detect early kidney damage by monitoring creatinine clearance rates and microalbumin excretion rates. The procedure for collecting the urine should be explained to the patient carefully. Written instructions should be supplied if the collection is to be performed at home. Collections are best obtained at a period of good control and normal activity, not during illness or menstruation; therefore the urine is often collected on an outpatient basis.

Ensure the correct containers are used for the collection. Ensure correct labelling of the specimen. The urine is tested for the presence of microalbuminuria, which is a predictor of kidney damage before overt proteinuria is detected by Multistix or Albustix.

Two new dipstix tests have recently become available for testing for microalbuminuria, and can be used in the ward situation. These are the:

● Micral test
● Microbumin test.

4.14   Further reading

Product information inserts.

Monitoring 3: additional biochemical assessment

In addition to blood and urine testing, diabetic control is assessed by:

(1) Regular weight checks.
(2) Regular physical examination, especially of:
   ● blood pressure (lying and standing to detect any postural drop which may indicate the presence of autonomic neuropathy)
   ● eyes (retina)
   ● cardiac status
   ● feet
   ● kidney function.
(3) Regular education about:
   ● diet
   ● self-monitoring techniques
   ● general diabetic knowledge
   ● changes to diabetes care as a result of research.

In addition special blood tests may be requested by the medical staff.

Normal ranges for the tests described will differ between laboratories depending on the assay method used.

4.15   Nursing responsibilities

(1) To have a basic knowledge of the tests in order to be able to explain them to the patient.
(2) To ensure the correct collection technique, appropriate amount of blood and correct tubes are used. Mix the sample by inverting the tube two or three times if an anticoagulant tube is required.

Vigorous shaking causes haemolysis of red blood cells.

---

(3) To ensure the specimen reaches the laboratory in the appropriate time span.
(4) To ensure results are available for medical evaluation.
(5) To know the effects of illness and stress on the results of the test.
(6) To ensure appropriate sterile blood collection technique.
(7) To ensure appropriate disposal of used equipment.
(8) To ensure fasting patients are given their medication and something to eat after completing the test.

4.16   Blood glucose

Venous glucose is measured to:

- Screen for diabetes.
- Monitor effectiveness of diabetic medication.
- Determine medication requirements.
- Evaluate diabetic control.
- Confirm high/low capillary glucose result.

Specimens should reach the laboratory within 30 minutes of collection or be refrigerated to prevent glycolysis occurring and consequent deterioration of the sample.

4.17   Glycosylated haemoglobin (HbA1c)

Circulating blood glucose attaches to the haemoglobin in the red blood cells and undergoes a chemical reaction whereby the glucose becomes permanently fixed to the haemoglobin (glycosylation). The glycosylated haemoglobin (HbA1c) can be measured and quantified to give an indication of metabolic control, in particular the average blood glucose concentration over the preceding 3 months.

It should be noted that:

- The rate of glycosylation of haemoglobin is influenced by chronic hyperglycaemia.
- HbA1c complements capillary blood glucose tests, and the clinical assessment of the patient.
- Fasting prior to obtaining the blood sample for HbA1c is not necessary.

People who experience frequent hypoglycaemic episodes may have satisfactory HbA1c results.

HbA1c results should be evaluated as part of the total clinical picture and not viewed in isolation.

There are several assay methods available for the determination of HbA1c values. Table 4.2 lists some factors which may affect HbA1c results.

4.18   Fructosamines

The fructosamines are a group of glycosylated blood and tissue proteins, and:

(1) They are dependent on blood glucose levels.
(2) They reflect average blood glucose levels within 3 weeks.
(3) They are useful for monitoring:
- diabetes during pregnancy
- initial response to diabetes medication
- patients with chronic anaemia
- patients with haemoglobinopathies.

Fructosamine results may be lower in patients with low serum albumin, cirrhosis of the liver or haemoglobinopathies.

Table 4.2   Non-glycaemic factors affecting results of glycosylated haemoglobin assays.

False high	False low
Chronic alcohol abuse	Abnormal haemoglobins
HbF	such as HbS, HbC, HbD
Hyperlipidaemia	Chronic blood loss
Hyperbilirubinaemia	Haemolysis
Renal failure	
Splenectomy	

4.19   Serum lipids

Serum lipids are usually elevated if the blood glucose is elevated. Three classes of lipids are measured:

(1) Cholesterol
(2) Triglycerides
(3) Lipoproteins:
- very low density lipoprotein (VLDL)
- low density lipoprotein (LDL)
- high density lipoprotein (HDL)

Fasting blood samples are most useful. Alcohol should not be consumed for 24 hours before the blood sample for serum lipid measurements is taken.

4.20   C-peptide

C-peptide is the connecting peptide which determines the folding of the two insulin chains during insulin production and storage in the pancreas. It splits off in the final stages and can be measured in the blood. It is used to measure pancreatic insulin production, to distinguish the type of diabetes if this is not clear in the clinical presentation. C-peptide is present in normal or elevated amounts in Type 2 diabetes, indicating that insulin is being produced and that diet and/or OHAs with exercise should achieve acceptable control.

● C-peptide will be absent or low in Type 1 diabetes.
● It is not changed by injections of insulin.
● Fasting results are most useful.

4.21 Creatinine clearance and urea

These are used to estimate renal function and nutritional status in relation to protein, especially during TPN and continuous ambulatory peritoneal dialysis (CAPD). An increase in the blood urea nitrogen (BUN) may indicate impaired renal function, however the BUN can also be increased if the patient is dehydrated, has internal bleeding or is on steroids. Anorexia, a low protein diet and fasting can lead to a decrease in urea.

Creatinine is a more sensitive marker of renal function. The serum creatinine is compared with the urine creatinine clearance rate over the same period of time. An increased serum creatinine indicates renal impairment. A significant rise may only occur when up to 50% of kidney function is lost. Creatinine is measured regularly to note *any* increase in the creatinine level.

4.22 Oral glucose tolerance Test (OGTT) (see section 1.5)

OGTT is used to confirm diabetes when fasting and random blood glucose results are equivocal, and:

● When there is a strong family history, especially during pregnancy.
● In the presence of the symptoms of diabetes, when all blood and urine glucose tests are normal.
● When the fasting and random blood glucose results are slightly elevated.

4.23 Further reading

Ismail, A. (1981) *Biochemical Investigations in Endocrinology and Diabetes Mellitus*. Academic Press, London.

Chapter 5
Dietary Aspects of Diabetic Nursing Care

5.1 Key points

- Promote good nutrition.
- Complex carbohydrate should be evenly spread throughout the day.
- Simple sugars should be avoided.
- The amount of fat should be decreased.
- The amount of salt should be decreased.
- Alcohol should be limited.
- Meals should be regular.

5.2 Introduction

The changing role of the nurse and the focus on the preventative aspects of health care mean that nurses have a responsibility to develop a knowledge of nutrition and its role in preventing disability and disease. It is integral to the adequate care of people with diabetes with respect to balancing energy intake, managing blood glucose and lipid levels and maintaining good nutrition.

Diseases such as diabetes, which are often associated with over-nutrition, may be prevented or ameliorated by avoiding excess weight. The recommended dietary guidelines, used in conjunction with the five food group plan for a nutritious diet, form the basis for dietary modification for diabetics. Diet is the mainstay and first line of treatment in the management of Type 2 diabetes.

An appropriate diet helps reduce the risk of developing diabetic complications, especially cardiovascular disease. The general dietary principles apply to all people with diabetes. Precise advice will vary according to individual lifestyle, eating habits, ethnic race and nutritional requirements. It is important that realistic targets be negotiated with the patient, particularly if weight control is necessary.

The effect of medications, fasting for procedures, and diarrhoea and vomiting on food absorption and consequently blood glucose levels is an important consideration. A basic screening tool to identify dietary and

nutritional characteristics should therefore be part of the nursing assessment and patient care plan, and allows appropriate referral to the dietitian.

Optimal nutritional care is best achieved by interaction between nursing
staff and the dietitian, their joint role effecting the most appropriate
management regime. Nursing staff have the greatest continuous contact
with the patient and so have an invaluable role in their nutritional
management by:

(1) Screening patients for gross nutritional states, such as underweight/
overweight.
(2) Screening patients' nutritional characteristics to identify potential
problems, e.g.:
   ● inappropriate/erratic eaters
   ● restricted eaters/overeaters
   ● those with domestic/financial/employment problems.
(3) Providing ongoing monitoring of patients on a meal-to-meal basis.

This information provides the basis from which nursing staff can quickly
and effectively refer patients to the dietitian, who can then support nursing
staff by:

● Setting goals of diet management consistent with life style and total
health care goals.
● Identifying possible nutritional problems.
● Identifying causes of possible problems.
● Counselling and educating the patient to best reduce the risks associated
with these problems.
● Supporting nursing and medical staff on an ongoing basis to ensure
most effective nutritional management has been achieved.

5.3   Method of screening for dietary characteristics and problems

5.3.1   Nutritional status

(1) Identify whether the person is overweight or underweight and whether
the person's health is affected by their weight status.
(2) Review any current haematological/biochemical measurements which
reflect the person's nutritional status (such as haemoglobin and serum
levels of albumin, folate and cholesterol).

5.3.2   Dietary characteristics

Determine:

- The regularity/irregularity of meals and/or snacks.
- Whether the person consumes foods and fluids containing refined sugar.
- Whether the person omits any of the major food groups.

If one or more problems are identified by the nurse, he/she can then refer the person to the dietitian for confirmation and further dietary analysis and advice.

5.4   Principles of dietary management for people with diabetes

In general the diet for people with diabetes should:

- Be high in complex carbohydrate (50–60% of total intake).
- Be low in fat (<10% of total energy value), especially saturated fat.
- Contain adequate protein (15% of total intake).
- Be free from simple sugar.
- Ensure a variety of food is eaten each day from each of the five food groups.
- Ensure that carbohydrate is consumed at each meal, especially for patients on insulin or diabetes medication.

The goals of dietary management are to:

- Improve the overall health of the patient by good nutrition.
- Attain optimal body weight.
- Attain acceptable lipid and blood glucose levels.
- Offer long-term support and education.
- Ensure normal growth and development in children.
- Decrease the risk of developing complications of diabetes.

5.4.1   Nursing responsibilities

(1) To assess dietary and nutritional characteristics and problems and refer to dietitian as required.
(2) To observe and, if necessary, record food intake, with particular reference to carbohydrate intake of patients on diabetic medication.
(3) To promote general dietary principles to patients in accordance with accepted policies and procedures.
(4) To ensure the meals and carbohydrate content are evenly spaced across the day.
(5) To ensure adequate carbohydrate intake for fasting patients, and those with diminished intake, to avoid hypoglycaemia.

Table 5.1 Drugs whose absorption may be modified by food.

Reduced absorption	Delayed absorption	Increased absorption
Aspirin	Aspirin	Diazepam
Cephalexin	Cefaclor	Dicoumarol
Erythromycin	Cephalexin	Erythromycin
Penicillin V and G	Cimetidine	Hydrochlorothiazide
Phenacetin	Digoxin	Metoprolol
Tetracycline	Indoprofen	Nitrofurantoin
Theophylline	Metronidazole	Propranolol

(6) To know that the absorption of some drugs may be modified by food, especially antibiotics, and their effectiveness may be diminished or increased. These drugs are detailed in Table 5.1.
(7) To observe for signs and symptoms of hyper- and hypoglycaemia, and correct same by appropriate administration of carbohydrate.

Inadequate nutrition can delay the healing process.

5.5 'Sugar-free' foods

'Sugar-free' usually refers to the sucrose content of foods. Other sugars are often used to sweeten foods labelled sugar-free (e.g. dextrose, fructose, maltose, lactose, galactose). They may not be appropriate for people with diabetes. Low calorie and artificially sweetened foods are generally recommended.

5.6 Non-nutritive sweeteners

Non-nutritive sweeteners are an acceptable alternative to sugar. For example:

● Saccharin
● Cyclamate
● Aspartame (Equal)
● Isomalt

However, the excessive use of these sugar substitutes is not recommended.
Sorbitol is another sweetener often used in diabetic products. It is not generally recommended because of its potential to cause diarrhoea in some patients. In addition, it has the same calorific value as glucose, and in

significant amounts can increase the blood glucose. Sorbitol is often used to sweeten biscuits and chocolates, manufactured for people with diabetes and sold by pharmacies and health food shops, etc. There are many varieties promoted. They are expensive and not recommended for people with diabetes.

5.7   Carbohydrate modified

Foods labelled 'carbohydrate modified' often have a high fat content and are not generally recommended for people with diabetes.

5.8   Dietetic foods

Foods labelled 'dietetic' may not be suitable for people with diabetes. It is important to encourage people to read food labels.

5.9   Alcohol

It is recommended that alcohol consumption be limited because of its potential to affect blood glucose and contribute to, or mask, hypoglycaemia (see Chapter 8). Sweet alcoholic drinks can lead to *hyper*glycaemia, while the alcohol itself leads to *hypo*glycaemia. Alcohol should *never* be consumed on an empty stomach.

Alcohol supplies considerable kilojoules and provides little or no nutritional value. In addition, alcohol clouds judgement and can lead to inappropriate decision making. Drunkenness can resemble hypoglycaemia and treatment of hypoglycaemia may be delayed.

5.10   'Exchanges' and 'portions'

Exchanges and portions are ways of measuring the carbohydrate content of the diet. They help to ensure an even distribution of carbohydrate when planning meals for individual patients. The difference between the two terms relates to the amount of carbohydrate measured. An exchange is equal to 15 g and a portion 10 g.

5.11   Glycaemic index

In the future the diabetic food plan may be based on the glycaemic index of foods. Glycaemic index is a method of comparing the effects of different carbohydrate containing foods on blood glucose.

5.12 Exercise/activity

Exercise has an important role in controlling the blood glucose and increasing overall fitness. It should be combined with a suitable diet. People commencing an exercise programme should first have a medical assessment. Before exercising they should check their blood glucose levels. It is important to make a gradual start to the exercise. Strenuous activity can cause hypoglycaemia; extra carbohydrate may be needed. The role of exercise in the management of diabetes is outlined in section 1.6.3.

5.13 Further reading

Australian Dietary Guidelines (1991) Australian Government Publications, Canberra.
Royal Australasian College of Physicians (1989) *Responsibility for Nutrition Diagnosis: A Report by the Nutrition Working Party of the Social Issues Committee of the Royal Australasian College of Physicians*. Smith-Gordon, Australia.
British Diabetic Association Report (1992) Dietary recommendations for people with diabetes, *Diabetic Medicine*, **9**, 189–202.

Chapter 6
Oral Hypoglycaemic Agents

6.1   Key points

- Administer 20 to 30 minutes before meals.
- Be aware of possible drug interactions.
- Presentation of hypoglycaemia may be atypical in people on oral hypoglycaemic agents.
- They are not insulin in oral form.

There are two types of oral hypoglycaemic agents (OHAs):

- Sulphonylureas
- Biguanides

Both classes of OHA improve the effectiveness of the person's own (endogenous) insulin. They don't contain insulin themselves. They should be used to supplement dietary measures. Excessive dosages are not recommended, nor are OHAs a substitute for proper dietary compliance. They are not prescribed for Type 1 diabetics nor during pregnancy.

6.2   Sulphonylureas

Sulphonylureas act by:

- Stimulating insulin secretion from the pancreatic beta cells.
- Increasing the effects of insulin at its receptor sites.
- Sensitizing hepatic glucose production to inhibition by insulin.

6.2.1   Possible side effects

(1) Hypoglycaemia may result due to oversecretion of insulin if the dose of the OHA is increased, food is delayed, meals are missed or activity is increased.
(2) Liver dysfunction.
(3) Nausea, vomiting.

(4) Various skin rashes.
(5) Increased appetite.
(6) *Rarely*, agranulocytosis and red cell aplasia may also occur.

Note: (2) to (6) are very uncommon. Sulphonylureas are contraindicated in pregnancy.

6.3   Biguanides

Biguanides act by:

- Impairing the absorption of glucose from the gut.
- Inhibiting gluconeogenesis (glucose production by the liver).
- Increasing glucose uptake into muscles and fat.
- Increasing the effects of insulin at receptor sites.
- Suppressing the appetite – mild effect.

Biguanides do not stimulate the production or release of insulin and therefore they do not produce hypoglycaemia.

6.3.1   Possible side effects

(1) In general, biguanides should not be used as a first line treatment because of the possibility of renal failure and lactic acidosis.
(2) Nausea and/or diarrhoea may occur in 10–15% of patients. Most patients tolerate biguanides if they are started at a low dose, the tablets are taken with or immediately after food and the dosage is increased gradually.
(3) Lactic acidosis may result if alcohol is consumed while taking biguanides.
(4) Biguanides should not be prescribed:
   - during pregnancy
   - for patients with chronic renal failure because they are excreted unchanged in the urine; lactic acidosis may occur in these patients.

The commonly available OHAs are listed in Table 6.1.

6.4   Drug interactions

Possible interactions between OHAs and commonly prescribed drugs are shown in Table 6.2.

Table 6.1 Currently available oral hypoglycaemic agents. (Adapted with permission from Bassaly, S. & Kydas, S. (1989) *Diatext, a Health Professional's Guide to Diabetes.* Ajay Printing, Melbourne.

Drug	Dose	Frequency	Possible side effects	Duration of action (DA)
(1) *Sulphonylureas*				
Chlorpropamide				
Diabinese 250 mg	125–500 mg	Single dose taken with,	Hypersensitivity	DA: 20–60 h
Promide 250 mg		or immediately after	Hypoglycaemia	
		food	Transient:	Peak: 5–7 h
			nausea	
			anorexia	
			vomiting	
			GI discomfort	
			May produce a disulfiram reaction with alcohol	
Glibenclamide				
Daonil 5 mg	2.5–20 mg	Up to 10 mg as a single dose	Side effects are rarely encountered, include:	DA: 6–12 h Peak: 6–8 h
Euglucon 5 mg		>10 mg in divided doses	nausea anorexia	
Glimel 5 mg		Taken with, or immediately before food	skin rashes Severe hypoglycaemia especially in elderly and those with renal dysfunction	
Glipizide				
Minidiab 5 mg	2.5–40 mg	Up to 15 mg as a single dose	GI disturbances Skin reactions	DA: Up to 24 h
		>15 mg in a twice daily dosage Taken immediately before meals	Hypoglycaemia (rare)	Peak 1–3 h
Tolbutamide				
Rastinon 0.5 g/1.0 g	0.5–3.0 g	1–3 times daily Taken immediately before food	Mild GI disturbances Hypoglycaemia (rare)	DA: 8–12 h Peak: 5–7 h
(2) *Biguanides*				
Metformin				
Diaformin 500 mg	0.5–1.5 g	1–3 times daily	GI disturbances	DA: 5–6 h
Diabex SR 500 mg	May be increased to	Taken with or	Tolerance may develop	
Glucophage 500 mg	3.0 g	immediately after food	Lactic acidosis may develop	

Table 6.2 Possible drug interactions with oral hypoglycaemic agents. (Adapted with permission from Bassaly, S. & Kydas, S. (1989) *Diatext, A Health Professional's Guide to Diabetes.* Ajay Printing, Melbourne.

Drug	Means of potentiation
(1) Drugs which may *Increase* the hypoglycaemic effect of sulphonylureas	
Sulphonamides Salicylates Warfarin Clofibrate Phenylbutazone	Displace sulphonylureas from protein binding sites
Coumarin derivatives Chloramphenicol Phenylbutazone	Inhibit/decrease hepatic metabolism
Probenecid Salicylates Tuberculostatics Tetracyclines	Delay urinary excretion
Sulphinpyrazone	Decreases plasma clearance
MAO inhibitors	Increases action by an unknown mechanism
(2) Drugs which may *inhibit* the hypoglycaemic effect of sulphonylureas	
Thiazides	Depress insulin release
Corticosteroids	Antagonize the action of insulin
Rifampicin	Decreases serum levels of tolbutamide
Glucagon	Stimulates the production of glucose from glycogen in the liver (used in the treatment of hypoglycaemia)
(3) Miscellaneous interactions	
Alcohol	Chronic alcohol abuse may stimulate the metabolism of sulphonylureas
Beta blockers	May mask tachycardia and other signs of hypoglycaemia
Thiazide diuretics	May cause hyperglycaemia

6.5 Combination of OHAs

There is no real benefit in using a combination of two sulphonylureas since they both act by the same mechanism. Sulphonylureas can be prescribed with biguanides for patients who have either primary or secondary failure with the sulphonylureas alone, especially if the patient is overweight.

Medication rounds should be planned so that OHAs are given with, or 20 to 30 minutes before, meals to decrease the risk of hypoglycaemia.

6.6   Combination of OHAs and insulin

In some patients a combination of insulin and sulphonylureas may help control the blood glucose. In these cases a small dose of intermediate/long-acting insulin given at bedtime may help control the blood glucose overnight, and thus reduce fasting hyperglycaemia in the morning. It is often easier to control the blood glucose during the day if the pre-breakfast test is <10 mmol/l.

6.7   Further reading

MS Publications (current edition) *Mims and Mims Annuals*. Griffin Press, Sydney.

Chapter 7
Insulin Therapy

7.1 Key points

- Clear insulin is drawn up before cloudy.
- Cloudy insulin must be mixed before drawing up.
- Check dose and time of administration.
- Give 20 to 30 minutes before a meal.
- Monitor blood glucose profile.
- Only clear (short-acting) insulin is given IV.

7.2 Basic insulin action

Insulin is a hormone secreted by the beta cells of the pancreas. Insulin synthesis and secretion are stimulated by an increase in the blood glucose level after meals. Insulin attaches to insulin receptors on cell membranes to facilitate the passage of glucose into the cell for utilization as fuel or for storage. Insulin also stimulates the storage of fatty acids and amino acids, and facilitates glycogen formation, and storage, in the liver. Therefore, an insulin deficiency results in altered protein, fat and carbohydrate metabolism.

7.3 Objectives of insulin therapy

(1) To achieve blood glucose levels within an acceptable individual range by replacing absent insulin secretion in Type 1 and supplementing insulin production in Type 2 diabetes.
(2) To approximate physiological insulin secretion.
(3) To avoid the consequences of too much insulin (hypoglycaemia) or too little insulin (hyperglycaemia).

7.4 Types of insulin available

There are a number of different brands of insulins available, e.g. Novo Nordisk, Eli Lilly. Insulin is derived from the pancreases of beef or pigs, or is manufactured by recombinant DNA technology (so-called 'human' insulin (HM)). Less commonly human insulin is made by modifying pork insulin.

The amino acid sequence of HM insulin is the same as that of insulin secreted by the beta cells of the human pancreas. HM is now the most commonly prescribed insulin regardless of the brand used. It is said to have a more rapid onset of action, shorter duration of action and decreased tendency to lead to the production of insulin antibodies, when compared to pork or beef insulin.

Human insulin does not come from humans.

Pork insulin is no longer generally available except in special circumstances as an individual patient usage (IPU) item, on the recommendation of an endocrinologist. Some older patients may still be taking beef insulin. Beef insulin is no longer generally prescribed for newly diagnosed patients.

Insulin preparations vary in their duration of action.

7.4.1   Short-acting insulin

This should be clear and colourless. Examples are:

- Actrapid
- Humulin R
- Velosulin
- Hypurin neutral (beef).

They begin to take effect in 20 to 30 minutes, and act for about 4 hours. They may be used:

- Alone two to four times daily.
- In combination with intermediate or long-acting insulins.
- As IV insulin infusions.

7.4.2   Intermediate-acting insulin

This must be mixed gently before use and should be milky after mixing. Examples are:

- Protophane
- Insulatard
- Lente
- Monotard
- Hypurin (beef)
- Isotard (beef)

They begin to act in 2 to 3 hours. The duration of action is 12 to 18 hours; the Lente and Monotard preparations, however, last for up to 22 hours. They may be used:

- In combination with short-acting insulin – this is the usual method.
- Alone for patients who are sensitive to short-acting insulin, or in combination with oral hypoglycaemic agents.

7.4.3 Long-acting insulin

This must be mixed before use and should be milky after mixing. Examples are:

- Ultralente
- Ultratard
- Protamine Zinc Insulin (beef)

They begin to act in 4 to 6 hours. The duration of action is 30 to 36 hours. Uses:

- As for intermediate-acting insulins.

7.4.4 Pre-mixed insulins

These contain both short- and intermediate-acting insulins in various combinations. They must be mixed before using. They do not allow for independent adjustment of short and intermediate components. Examples are:

- Mixtard (30/70%)
- Mixtard (50/50%)
- Mixtard (15/85%)

They may be used by:

- Patients who do not require perfect control.
- Those who have difficulty mixing insulins (e.g. the elderly).

7.5 Storage of insulin

Store unopened vials in the refrigerator at 2–8°C.

Do not freeze. Check expiry date. Discard if outdated.

7.6   Injection site and administration

Insulin should be given 20 to 30 minutes before the meal. The abdomen is the preferred site; upper arms, thighs and buttocks can also be used. Injection sites must be rotated.

Pinch up a fold of skin. Push the needle into the skin at right angles. Inject the insulin. Remove the needle and apply pressure to the site. Document dose and time of the injection. Check injection sites for swelling, lumps, pain or leakage of insulin.

Tips

● If insulin tends to leak after injection release the skin fold before injecting. Pressure from holding the skin fold sometimes forces the insulin back out of the needle track. Withdraw the syringe quickly.
● Long-acting and pre-mixed insulins for insulin pens must be mixed gently before administration.

Instructions about how to draw up and administer insulin appear in Chapter 18.

7.7   Mixing short- and long-acting insulins

7.7.1   General points

Mixing short- and long-acting insulins before injection may have the effect of diminishing the short-acting peak, which is more marked when there is substantially more long-acting insulin in the mixture (as is usually the case), especially if the insulin is:

● Left to stand for a long time before use.
● Mixed with insulin zinc suspensions (Lente).

If a short-acting insulin contains a phosphate buffer, it should never be mixed with an insulin zinc suspension, which contains acetate buffer, because it has the effect of making the Lente and Ultralente insulin short-acting.

7.8   Common insulin regimes

7.8.1   Daily injection

A combination of short- and long-acting insulin usually given before breakfast. Premixed insulins such as Mixtard may be used. Daily regimes are commonly used for:

- Elderly people.
- Those not willing to have more than one injection.

They are *not* recommended for young IDDM.

7.8.2 Twice daily regime

A combination of short- and longer-acting insulin is usually given before breakfast and before tea. Pre-mixed insulins may be used. This allows more flexibility in adjusting doses. Usually two-thirds of the total dose is given in the morning and one-third in the evening.

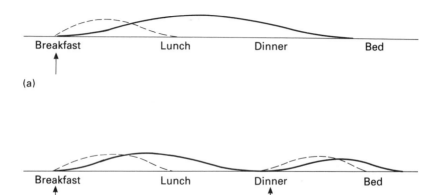

(a)

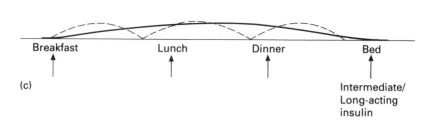

(c)

Fig. 7.1 Diagrammatic representation of insulin action showing (a) daily, (b) BD and (c) basal bolus regimes.

Note: The broken line depicts short-acting insulin, the unbroken line intermediate/long-acting insulin. The arrows indicate the time of injection.

7.8.3 Basal bolus regime

Basal bolus regimes simulate the normal pattern of insulin secretion. Bolus injections of short-acting insulin are given before each meal. The longer-acting insulin is given before bed to supply the basal insulin requirement. This regime offers more flexibility in insulin dose adjustment and meal times, and therefore lifestyle is less restricted. The amount of insulin given at each dose is usually small, therefore the likelihood of hypoglycaemia is reduced. It is commonly used for young people with Type 1 diabetes.

Insulin pens which are discreet and portable are often used for basal bolus regimes (see Chapter 18). Patients should continue to use their pens in hospital. Figure 7.1 is a diagrammatic representation of insulin action showing daily, BD and basal bolus regimes.

7.9 Continuous subcutaneous insulin infusion (CSII)

Insulin pumps deliver insulin continuously via the subcutaneous route (basal) with a bolus dose given before meals. They are not commonly used and are expensive. The pump is worn most of the time and may not be acceptable to many people.

The choice of regime depends on personal patient preference, the degree of blood glucose control aimed for, and the patient's ability to monitor blood glucose. Many factors can influence insulin absorption and consequently blood glucose; some of these factors are shown in Table 7.1.

Table 7.1 Factors affecting insulin absorption.

Accelerated	Delayed
Exercise	Low body temperature
High temperature	Poor circulation
Massage round injection site	Smoking
Depth of injection	Long-acting insulins

7.10 Sliding scale and top-up regimes

A sliding scale of insulin refers to a regime where the amount of insulin given varies according to the blood glucose result. An example of a sliding scale is given in section 7.11. Sliding scales are often used in conjunction with intravenous insulin infusions, or when managing patients pre- and post-operatively.

Sliding scales are not generally useful for stabilizing newly diagnosed patients, because:

- Blood glucose levels are often erratic.
- They delay the establishment of an appropriate insulin dose.
- They adjust insulin according to blood glucose only, and do not take into account other factors affecting control, such as diet.

It is preferable to monitor the blood glucose over 24–48 hours and adjust the insulin according to the emerging pattern and the daily, BD or basal bolus insulin regime chosen. Top-up doses of insulin may be required if the blood glucose is high or moderate/large ketones are present. Often extra short-acting insulin is added to the next due dose of insulin.

The dose of insulin for the next day may need to be reviewed and assessed by the doctor. Sliding and top-up scales are generally only used in hospital or managing unwell patients at home in special circumstances.

7.11   Intravenous insulin infusions

The IV route is preferred for very ill patients because the absorption of insulin is more reliable than from poorly perfused muscle and fat tissue. Absorption may be erratic in these patients, especially if they are hypotensive. The aims of the insulin infusion are to:

- Switch off liver's conversion of glycogen and fatty acids to glucose and therefore avoid hyperglycaemia.
- Prevent utilization of fatty acids and therefore limit ketone formation.
- Decrease peripheral resistance to insulin.
- Gradually decrease the blood glucose concentration to 10–12 mmol/l without subjecting the patient to hypoglycaemia.

The medication order for the infusion must be clearly and legibly written on the treatment sheet. Insulin doses for IV insulin infusions are usually 0.1 U/kg/h. Sometimes an initial bolus of 5-10 units will be given. In general a low dose infusion such as this has been shown to reduce the blood glucose, ketosis and acidosis as effectively as high dose regimes, without the added risk of hypoglycaemia. The rate at which the insulin is to be administered should be written in ml/h and units to be delivered. Several protocols exist; the following is one example.

The infusion rate is adjusted according to the patient's blood glucose results (tested 2 hourly). This is basically a sliding scale of insulin. For example:

Blood glucose (mmol/l)	Insulin (U/h)
0–6	0
6–11	1
11–15	2
15–19	3
>19	4
>24	Notify doctor

The insulin order and blood glucose results should be reviewed regularly.

7.11.1   Preparing the insulin solution to be infused

Two people should check and make up the solution according to the medication order and hospital protocols.

Only clear short-acting insulin is used for insulin infusions.
Solutions must be gently mixed and if not in haemaccel discard the first 50 ml through the giving set (to allow for insulin binding to the plastic).

It has been well documented that insulin binds to plastic IV containers and tubing. Several methods have been used to minimize the binding. They include:

- Addition of human serum albumin to the solution.
- Flushing the infusion set with the insulin solution to saturate the binding sites before connecting it to the patient.

All solutions must be discarded after 24 hours.

7.12   Uses of insulin infusions

7.12.1   General use (during surgical procedures)

Insulin is added to 4% dextrose in $\frac{1}{5}$ normal saline or 5% dextrose. The infusion is often given via *burette* at 120 ml/h (i.e. 8 hourly rate; see previous example scale). Monitor blood glucose 2 to 3 hourly and review with medical staff *regularly*.

7.12.2   Special needs

- Open heart surgery.
- Ketoacidosis.
- Hyperosmolar coma.
- Intensive care unit (ICU) situations.

These situations always require the use of a controlled rate infusion pump

(IMED pump or syringe pump) to ensure accurate administration of the insulin. It is often necessary to limit the amount of fluid administered to avoid cerebral oedema. Standard regimes include:

(1) Haemaccel 100 ml + 100 U Actrapid = 1 U/1 ml, used in ICU and administered via IMED.
(2) Haemaccel 500 ml + 100 U Actrapid = 1 U/5 ml via IMED.

People who are insulin-resistant, such as those who:

● Have liver disease.
● Are on steroid therapy.
● Are obese.
● Have a serious infection.

may require more insulin, i.e. a high dose infusion (more units per hour).

Subcutaneous insulin must be given prior to removing the infusion and the patient must be eating and drinking normally to avoid excursions in blood glucose concentrations.

7.13   Risks associated with insulin infusions

● Hypoglycaemia.
● Cardiac arrhythmias.
● Sepsis at IV site.
● Fluid overload.

7.14   Factors affecting insulin delivery via infusion

● Accuracy of system (including blood glucose testing).
● Stability of solution.
● Circulatory insufficiency.

7.15   Mistakes associated with insulin infusions

(1) If insulin is added to the burette rather than the bag of IV fluid, refilling the burette from the bag results in no insulin being administered. Therefore hyperglycaemia results.
(2) Incorrect amount of insulin added to bag/burette. This may be a result of inadequate checking of dose, not using an insulin syringe or failing to check illegible medical orders.

(3) The insulin infusion is often run at the same time as other intravenous fluids (e.g. 4% dextrose in $^1/_5$ normal saline). The most common method is to infuse the different fluids through the one IV cannula using a three-way adaptor ('octopus').

Usually the dextrose or saline is running at a faster rate than the insulin infusion. Problems can arise if there is a complete or partial blockage of the cannula. The force of gravity pushing the fluid toward the vein can actually cause the dextrose/saline to flow back up the slower flowing insulin line resulting in high blood glucose levels. Figure 7.2 depicts the result of a blockage in the IV cannula and three-way adaptor, during the concurrent administration of insulin and dextrose/saline.

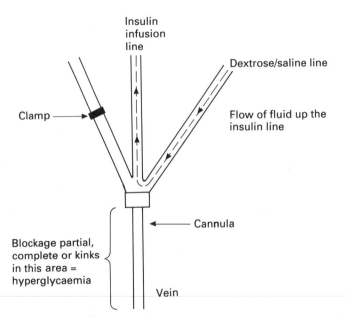

Fig. 7.2 Possible results of a blockage in the IV cannula and three-way adaptor during the concurrent administration of insulin and dextrose/saline.

Action
If hyperglycaemia occurs check:

● That the tubing and adaptors are patent.
● That insulin has been added to the burette/bag.
● That the amount of insulin added is correct.
● Possible sources of infection.

7.16 Further reading

Galloway, J.A. (1988) Chemistry and clinical use of insulin. In *Diabetes Mellitus* (ed. J.A. Galloway), Chapter 7. Eli Lilly, Indianapolis.

Metheny, N.M. (1992) *Fluid and Electrolyte Balance*, Chapter 21. Lippincott, Philadelphia.

Novo Nordisk (1991) *Insulin and Diabetes: Reference Manual for Health Professionals*.

Chapter 8
Hypoglycaemia

8.1 Key points

- Treat promptly.
- Treat adequately.
- Monitor recovery.
- Seek cause.
- Document episode.
- Educate patient.

8.2 Introduction

Some nursing staff find it difficult to distinguish between hypoglycaemia and hyperglycaemia. Many journal articles and reference texts discuss these topics together under headings such as 'The diabetic comas', which often adds to the confusion. A state of hypoglycaemia or hyperglycaemia (including ketosis) can occur without the patient being comatose or unconscious. The only conclusive method of distinguishing between the two is to perform a blood glucose test. Results of <3 mmol/l in people taking insulin or oral hypoglycaemic agents indicate hypoglycaemia.

My preference has been to consider these two very different entities requiring different management in separate chapters.

8.3 Definition of hypoglycaemia

Hypoglycaemia occurs when the blood glucose falls low enough to cause signs and symptoms. It is usually defined as a blood glucose level of <3.0 mmol/l in diabetic patients treated with insulin or oral hypoglycaemic agents.

Diabetic patients who are managed by diet alone do not require treatment of low blood glucose levels.

Table 8.1 Signs and symptoms of hypoglycaemia.

Sympathetic*	Neuroglucopenic†
Weakness	Headache
Sweating	Hypothermia
Tachycardia	Visual disturbances
Palpitations	Mental dullness
Tremor	Confusion
Nervousness	Amnesia
Irritability	Seizures
Tingling of mouth and fingers	Coma
Hunger	

*Caused by increased activity of the autonomic nervous system; triggered by a rapid fall in blood glucose
†Caused by decreased activity of the central nervous system; because of very low blood glucose.

Nausea and vomiting may occur but are unusual.

Age, sex and associated medical conditions (liver disease, cerebrovascular disease and autonomic neuropathy) and the rate at which the glucose falls may influence the development and recognition of symptoms. In general a rapid decrease in blood glucose results in the development of the classic symptoms of hypoglycaemia described in Table 8.1. The classic presentation is more likely to occur in insulin-treated patients.

8.4 Recognition of hypoglycaemia

Some, or all, of the signs and symptoms listed in Table 8.1 may be present. Symptoms may be less obvious in people treated with OHAs, where hypoglycaemia tends to develop much more slowly and the classic signs may not be present. The patient may complain of lethargy, tiredness or dizziness. Severe cases may present as cerebrovascular accident resulting in delayed treatment. The hypoglycaemia may be prolonged and may recur or become chronic.

8.5 Counter-regulatory hormonal response to hypoglycaemia

The brain requires 120–140 g glucose per day to function normally. When the blood glucose falls below normal the body releases hormones to

Table 8.2   The counter-regulatory hormonal response to hypoglycaemia.

Hormone	Action
Glucagon	Increased glucose output (glycogenolysis)
Epinephrine and norepinephrine	Enhanced glycogenolysis in liver and muscle Enhanced gluconeogenesis Decreased insulin secretion Causes many of the signs and symptoms of hypoglycaemia (sympathetic response; see Table 8.1)
Cortisol	Mobilizes substrate for gluconeogenesis
Growth hormone	Acts with cortisol and epinephrine to inhibit peripheral glucose utilization
	The net result is increased blood glucose

counteract the effects of hypoglycaemia. This is known as the counter-regulatory response. Glycogen stores are liberated and new glucose is formed from precursors. The hormones released are shown in Table 8.2, along with their resultant action, the nett result being an increase in blood glucose.

8.6   Objectives of care

To be alert to the possibility of hypoglycaemia in all patients on insulin or OHAs, and should it occur to:

(1) Immediately raise blood glucose levels.
(2) Maintain blood glucose levels within the acceptable range of 4–10 mmol/l.
(3) Ascertain the cause of the hypoglycaemic episode.
(4) Limit further episodes of hypoglycaemia.
(5) Allay fear and anxiety.
(6) Prevent trauma occurring as a result of hypoglycaemia.

8.7   Treatment

Rapid treatment is important.

8.7.1   Conscious patient

Test and record the blood glucose level.

First: give quick-acting sugar to raise the blood glucose immediately, e.g.:

3 level teaspoons sugar in $\frac{1}{2}$ cup water, tea or coffee
or   1 cup orange juice
or $\frac{1}{2}$ regular soft drink (*not low calorie* (joule))
or   proprietary glucose preparation such as glucose gels/tablets.

Second: follow with long-acting carbohydrate to maintain blood glucose until the next meal time, e.g.:

$\frac{1}{2}$ sandwich
or   2 to 4 dry biscuits
or   1 piece of fruit
or   2 plain sweet biscuits.

Check blood glucose in one hour then as necessary. The next dose of insulin or OHA is not usually withheld following a mild hypoglycaemic episode.

8.7.2   Impaired conscious state

Note: do not give anything by mouth.

(1) Place patient on side.
(2) Clear airway.
(3) One nurse notify doctor.
(4) Second nurse test blood glucose level and confirm with chemical pathology (i.e. urgent glucose).
(5) Assemble glucagon and IV tray containing 50% dextrose. (Dextrose may be given by minijet). Instructions for glucagon administration appear in section 8.14.
(6) Give complex carbohydrate when consciousness returns. The patient may still be confused and may need to be reminded to chew and swallow.
(7) Repeat fingerprick in one hour then as necessary, but not less than 4 hourly.

Patient should be monitored for at least 36 hours. Ascertain the time and dose for the next insulin injection/OHA dose.

8.7.3   In both cases

Recovery should be rapid.

(1) Record episode and blood glucose level on diabetic chart and in patient unit record.
(2) Monitor progress/recovery from episode.
(3) Look for cause of hypoglycaemia (e.g. meal delayed or missed, inadequate intake of carbohydrate, unaccustomed activity, excessive medication).
(4) Reassure the patient.
(5) Ensure patient has an understanding of causes and management of hypoglycaemia (refer to diabetes educator).

8.8   Nocturnal hypoglycaemia

The blood glucose may drop during the night (around 2 to 3 AM) and hypoglycaemia can go unnoticed by the patient.

8.8.1   Indicators

- Night sweats.
- Nightmares.
- Unaccustomed snoring.
- Morning lethargy.
- Headaches.
- Depression.
- High blood glucose before breakfast (Somogyi effect).
- Morning ketonuria.

The Somogyi effect refers to pre-breakfast hyperglycaemia following an overnight hypoglycaemic episode.

If any of the above occur the blood glucose should be measured at 2 to 3 AM over several nights to establish if nocturnal hypoglycaemia is occurring. The insulin is then adjusted accordingly by decreasing the morning long-acting dose for those on a daily insulin, the afternoon long-acting dose for those on BD insulin or basal bolus regimes.

The Somogyi effect should be distinguished from another condition resulting in morning hyperglycaemia, the 'dawn phenomenon'. The dawn phenomenon refers to a situation where insulin requirements and blood glucose concentration increase between 5 AM and 8 AM. It occurs in up to 75% of diabetic patients. Treatment consists of *increasing* the insulin dose.

8.9   Chronic hypoglycaemia

In elderly people on OHAs hypoglycaemia may become chronic and present as failing mental function, personality changes or disordered behaviour. Accurate monitoring of the blood glucose levels is important to detect chronic hypoglycaemia.

8.10   Relative hypoglycaemia

People who are accustomed to high blood glucose levels for long periods of time may experience the symptoms of hypoglycaemia at normal blood glucose levels. In general it is not necessary to treat the symptoms once the blood glucose is recorded, but support and education are necessary until the patient adapts to the new blood glucose range.

8.11   Drug interactions

Some commonly prescribed drugs may interact with the sulphonylurea prescribed to control the blood glucose, increasing the possibility of hypoglycaemia (see Table 8.3).

Table 8.3   Commonly prescribed drugs which may increase the hypoglycaemic effect of sulphonylurea agents.

Drugs	Means of potentiation
Sulphonamides Salicylates Warfarin Clofibrate Phenylbutazone	Displaces sulphonylureas from protein binding sites
Coumarin derivatives Chloramphenicol Phenylbutazone	Inhibits/decreases hepatic metabolism of the Sulphonylurea
Probenecid Salicylates Tuberculostatics Tetracyclines	Delays urinary excretion of the Sulphonylurea
MAO inhibitors	Increases action by an unknown mechanism

8.12   Patients most at risk of hypoglycaemia

(1) Those taking insulin or OHAs.
(2) Those with renal, kidney or hepatic disease.
(3) Those with long-standing diabetes who no longer recognize sympathetic warning signs.
(4) Those with autonomic neuropathy.
(5) People fasting for a procedure/surgery.
(6) People with diarrhoea and vomiting.
(7) Those with an impaired conscious state.
(8) Those sedated or on narcotic infusions.
(9) Those on long-acting diabetic medications (e.g. chlorpropamide, Ultratard).
(10) The elderly.
(11) Those beginning an exercise/diet regime.

Alcohol may also cause hypoglycaemia, particularly if food is not eaten at the same time. The hypoglycaemia can occur hours after consuming alcohol.

8.13   Psychological effects of hypoglycaemia

Hypoglycaemia is feared and hated by many people with diabetes and often underrated by health professionals. Commonly expressed concerns are:

● Loss of control of the situation.
● Reminder that they have diabetes.
● Losing face and making a fool of themselves.
● Sustaining brain damage.
● Dying.

Hypoglycaemia can lead to decreased confidence in the ability to cope. It is not unknown for people to run their blood glucose high to avoid 'having a hypo'. They may then be termed 'non-compliant' and placed in a conflict situation. Support and understanding are vital.

8.14   Guidelines for the administration of glucagon

Glucagon is a hormone produced by the alpha cells of the pancreas which acts on the liver to release glucose. Glucagon is available in a single dose pack containing one vial of glucagon hydrochloride powder (1 mg) and a glass syringe prefilled with sterile water (water for injections).

8.14.1   Indication

Glucagon is used to treat severe hypoglycaemic reactions in diabetic people treated with insulin or OHAs.

8.14.2   Instructions for use

(1) Individual patients must be assessed to determine dose and route of administration. Glucagon is given according to body weight and muscle bulk (intramuscular or subcutaneously). The buttock is the ideal injection site.
(2) The intravenous route may be the preferred route in profound hypoglycaemia to ensure rapid absorption.
(3) Glucagon should be used soon after reconstitution. Do not use if reconstituted solution is not clear and colourless.

8.14.3   Dosage

● Adults and children of weight >25 kg full dose (1/1)
● Children of weight <25 kg half dose (1/2).

Glucagon may be repeated, however repeated injections can cause nausea, making subsequent food intake difficult.

8.15   Further reading

Alberti, K.G.M.M. (1988) Diabetic emergencies. In *Diabetes Mellitus*, (ed. J. Galloway), pp. 253–360. Eli Lilly, Indianapolis.
McCarthy, J. (1979) Somogyi effect: Managing blood glucose rebound. *Nursing*, 9, 39–41.
National Health and Medical Research Council (1991) *Hypoglycaemia and Diabetes*. Australian Government Printers, Canberra.

Chapter 9
Stabilization of Diabetes

9.1 Key points

- In many cases ambulatory stabilization is preferred.
- Encourage independence.
- Allow patient to perform own self-care tasks.

Stabilization of diabetes refers to the process of achieving an optimal blood glucose range, appropriate diabetes knowledge and management of diabetic complications, either acute or chronic. Stabilization may occur at initial diagnosis of diabetes, when a change of treatment is indicated (transfer from oral agents to insulin therapy), and for antenatal care.

In many cases stabilization of diabetes can be achieved without admitting the patient to hospital. This process is known as ambulatory stabilization. Ambulatory stabilization requires specialized staff, specific protocols and ample time if it is to be successful. It can result in considerable cost benefits, and reduces the stress associated with a hospital admission.

However, some patients will continue to be admitted to hospital for stabilization of their diabetes.

9.2 Stabilization of diabetes in hospital

Patients admitted to improve their metabolic control (stabilization) are not generally ill and should be encouraged to:

- Keep active.
- Wear clothes instead of pyjamas.
- Perform diabetes self-care tasks (blood glucose monitoring and insulin administration).

They will require support, encouragement and consistent advice. The time spent in hospital should be kept to a minimum.

9.2.1 Nursing responsibilities

(1) Inform the appropriate staff about the admission (diabetes educator, dietitian).
(2) Assess the patient carefully (refer to Chapter 2).
(3) Monitor blood and urine glucose according to protocols; for example, 7 AM, 11 AM, 4 PM and 9 PM.
(4) Supervise and assess the patient's ability to test their own blood glucose and/or administer insulin.
(5) Ensure diabetes knowledge is assessed and updated: new learning needs may include insulin techniques, sharps disposal, hypoglycaemia and home management during illness.
(6) TPR daily, or every second day.
(7) BP, lying and standing daily.
(8) Ensure all blood samples, urine collections and special tests are performed accurately. The opportunity is often taken to perform a comprehensive complication screen while the patient is in hospital. This may include ECG, eye referral, 24-hour urine collection for creatinine and microalbumin.
(9) Ensure the patient has supplies of test strips, lancets, syringes, etc. before discharge and that the appropriate follow-up appointments have been made.

9.3 Ambulatory stabilization

The types of ambulatory services provided for people with diabetes include:

● Diabetes education.
● Commencement on medication (oral agents, insulin).
● Complication screening and assessment.
● Blood glucose testing.
● Consultations with dietitian, diabetes educator or diabetes specialist.
● Clinical assessment.

The specific protocol and policy of the employing institution should be followed and all contacts and telephone advice documented. The following is an example protocol for insulin stabilization on an ambulatory basis.

9.3.1 Objectives of ambulatory stabilization onto insulin

Short-term objectives
(1) To reassure and allay the fear that everything about diabetes must be learned at once.

(2) To establish trust between the patient and the diabetes team.
(3) To gradually normalize blood glucose.
(4) To teach the 'survival skills' necessary for the patient to be safe at home:
  - insulin drawing up and administration
  - blood glucose monitoring
  - recognizing and treating hypoglycaemia
  - how to obtain advice – contact telephone number.

Long-term objectives
The aim in the long term is for the patient to:

(1) Accept diabetes as part of life, and recognize their part in the successful management of the diabetes (lifestyle should be modified as little as possible).
(2) Be able to make appropriate changes in insulin doses, carbohydrate intake and activity to maintain acceptable blood glucose levels.
(3) Be able to maintain an acceptable range of blood glucose, HbA1c and cholesterol.
(4) Be able to maintain a healthy weight range.
(5) Modify risk factors to prevent or delay the onset of the long-term complications of diabetes and therefore the need for hospital admissions.
(6) Attend regular medical/education appointments.
(7) Receive ongoing support and encouragement from the diabetes team.

9.3.2 Rationale for choosing ambulatory stabilization

Stabilization onto insulin on an outpatient basis is preferred if possible for the following reasons:

(1) To avoid the 'sick role' which can be associated with a hospital admission.
(2) It is cost effective, i.e. does not require a hospital bed.
(3) It involves less time away from work and usual activity for the patient, who can therefore be stabilized according to his/her usual routine, rather than hospital routines and food.
(4) To encourage self-reliance and confidence.
(5) Outpatient stabilization is labour-intensive, however unhurried time is necessary if the process is to be successful.

9.3.3 Criteria for patient selection for ambulatory stabilization

The patient must be:

- Able to attend daily for a period of about 3 to 5 days; in some cases twice daily visits may be necessary.
- Physically and mentally capable of performing blood glucose monitoring and insulin administration, or have assistance to do so.

In addition, some social/family support is helpful.

9.3.4 The process of stabilization

(1) It should involve members of the diabetes team as appropriate.
(2) Communication, especially between the doctor, educator, dietitian and patient, is essential.
(3) Patients should be assessed on an individual basis, so that appropriate education goals and blood glucose range can be determined. The insulin regime will depend on individual requirements.
(4) Formal teaching days should not include weekends or public holidays unless staff are available.
(5) Adequate charting and documentation of progress should be recorded after each session (blood glucose results, ability to manage insulin technique, goals of management).

Patient Instruction Sheet 3 is an example protocol for ambulatory stabilization onto insulin.

9.4 Further reading

National Health and Medical Research Council (1991) *The Role of Ambulatory Services in the Management of Diabetes*. Document No. 1. Australia.

PATIENT CARE SHEET 3:
PROTOCOL FOR AMBULATORY STABILIZATION
ONTO INSULIN

SUGGESTED PROTOCOL

**These are guidelines only and should be
modified to suit individual needs**

Day One

Aim to commence at 7.30-8 am. The length of stay will depend on the patient and the insulin regime decided upon. If a full day stay is envisaged a 2-3 hour break in the middle is usually necessary.

(1)   Introduce the diabetes team and area facilities.

(2)   Test blood glucose.

(3)   Insulin dose/frequency is determined in consultation with the doctor.

(4)   Educator draws up and gives the insulin and explains the procedure to the patient.

(5)   Breakfast.

(6)   It is important to encourage the patient to discuss his/her feelings about diabetes and to assess current diabetes knowledge, learning capacity and social situation.

Education Goals

(1)   To give a basic explanation of what diabetes is and what is an acceptable blood glucose range.

(2)   To explain the reason for instituting insulin therapy.

(3)   To explain the effects of insulin on blood glucose levels, ie. insulin action and the role of long and short-acting insulin in control of blood glucose levels.

PATIENT CARE SHEET 3 *contd*

(4) To explain insulin technique:

- drawing up

- sites for injection

- expiry dates of insulin bottles

- care and storage

- appropriate sharps disposal.

(5) To explain why insulin must be given by injection, and allow patient to handle a syringe and insulin bottles and practise the drawing up of insulin.

(6) To explain hypoglycaemia:

- recognition of low blood glucose levels symptoms

- causes and prevention

- effective management

- patient should carry carbohydrate for "emergencies".

(7) Blood glucose monitoring should be encouraged, to provide feedback to the patient and enable him/her to telephone in the afternoon with a result if necessary. The role of monitoring should be explained as well as the timing of testing and how to record results.

(8) Basic introduction to a food plan: role of carbohydrate in blood glucose control and the need for regular meals.

(9) If on twice daily insulin, the injection and dinner may be given before the patient leaves, or the insulin can be drawn up for the patient to give at home.

(10) Explain and enrol the patient in the National Diabetes Supply Scheme[*] Give diabetes booklets and brochures as appropriate.

(11) Ensure patient has starter kit for insulin and monitoring and knows how and where to obtain future supplies.

Point (10) above: the National Diabetes Supply Scheme only applies in Australia.

PATIENT CARE SHEET 3 *contd*

Day Two

(1)   Patient comes at 8 am and stays 2-3 hours. If on twice daily insulin the patient may return in the afternoon or give own dose after telephoning staff with blood glucose result; depending on accuracy of insulin technique.

(2)   Test blood glucose.

(3)   Insulin dose is determined (consultation with doctor may be necessary). Patient to draw up and give own injection under supervision. Document in patient record.

Education Goals

(1)   Revision of day one and answer any questions the patient may have.

(2)   Detailed revision of blood glucose monitoring and insulin technique.

(3)   Explanation of renal threshold and role of urine testing, especially with regard to testing for ketones in IDDM.

(4)   Detailed food plan and revision of role of carbohydrate and sweeteners: with dietitian if possible.

Days Three, Four and Five

As for day two. Revision of previous day's information and questions answered. Patient should be testing own blood glucose and giving own insulin injection, under supervision.

PATIENT CARE SHEET 3 *contd*

Education Goals

(1) Discuss how to manage illness at home, in relation to:

- who to contact
- effects of illness on blood glucose
- emergency diet
- monitoring and recording of blood glucose and urine ketones
- adjusting/continuing insulin
- need to rest.

(2) Discuss precautions to be taken relating to driving, work, etc.

(3) Discuss the role of exercise/activity in controlling blood glucose levels.

(4) Prescriptions for insulin, test strips, syringes, etc. should be finalised.

(5) Complete food plan.

(6) Encourage patient to wear some form of identification.

(7) Ensure that patient has a contact telephone number and knows who to contact for advice.

(8) Provide appropriate follow-up appointments for doctor, educator according to patient needs.

(9) Provide ongoing individual teaching as required.

(10) Ensure patient knows about other services available for people with diabetes, eg. Diabetes Associations.

(11) Arrange for consultation with family if necessary.

Chapter 10

Hyperglycaemia, Diabetic Ketoacidosis (DKA) and Hyperosmolar Coma

10.1 Key points

- Be prepared.
- Meticulous attention to detail.
- Monitor rehydration closely.
- Gradually decrease blood glucose.
- Monitor urine, ketone clearance.
- Educate patient.

10.2 Hyperglycaemia

Hyperglycaemia refers to an elevated blood glucose level (>10 mmol/l) due to a relative or absolute insulin deficiency. The symptoms of hyperglycaemia usually occur when the blood glucose is persistently above 15 mmol/l; see section 1.3. The cause of the hyperglycaemia should be sought, and corrected to avoid the development of diabetic ketoacidosis (DKA) or hyperosmolar coma. Hyperglycaemia, DKA and hyperosmolar coma are often referred to as short-term complications of diabetes.

10.3 Diabetic ketoacidosis (DKA)

Diabetic ketoacidosis is a life-threatening complication of diabetes. The basic pathophysiology consists of a relative or absolute insulin deficiency. Glucose is unable to enter the cells and accumulates in the blood. Insulin deficiency also leads to the metabolism of fats with the formation of free fatty acids and subsequently ketone bodies. Protein catabolism also occurs and forms the substrates for gluconeogenesis, further increasing the blood glucose. It usually only occurs in Type 1 patients, but may occur in Type 2 people with severe infections or metabolic stress.

Diabetic ketoacidosis is characterized by hyperglycaemia, osmotic diuresis, metabolic acidosis, glycosuria, ketonuria and dehydration. The definition by laboratory results is blood glucose >17 mmol/l; ketonaemia, (ketone bodies) >3 mmol/l; acidosis, pH <7.30 and bicarbonate <15 mEq/l.

The signs, symptoms and precipitating factors for DKA are shown in Table 10.1, while Fig. 10.1 outlines the physiology, the signs and symptoms which occur as a result of decreased utilization of glucose and the biochemical manifestations found on blood testing.

Table 10.1 Signs, symptoms and precipitating factors in diabetic ketoacidosis (DKA).

Symptoms and signs	Precipitating factors
Thirst	(1) Newly diagnosed IDDM (20–30%)
Polyuria	(2) Omission of insulin therapy
Fatigue	(3) Inappropriate dose reduction
Weight loss	(4) Relative insulin deficiency
Nausea and vomiting	(a) Acute illness:
Abdominal pain	Infection (50% of cases)
Muscle cramps	Myocardial infarction
Tachycardia	Trauma, acute stress
Kussmauls respirations	Cerebrovascular accident
	(b) Endocrine disorders (rare):
	Hyperthyroidism
	Pheochromocytoma
	Acromegaly
	Cushing's disease
	(c) Drugs:
	Cortisone
	Thiazide diuretics

10.3.1 Late signs, i.e. severe DKA

The initial signs and symptoms of DKA (polyuria, polydipsia, lethargy and Kussmauls respirations) are an attempt by the body to compensate for the acidosis. If treatment is delayed the body eventually decompensates. Signs of decompensation (late signs) include:

● Warm, dry skin.
● Hypothermia.
● Hypoxia and decreased conscious state.
● Decreased renal output (oliguria).
● Decreased respirations – absence of Kussmauls respirations.
● Bradycardia.

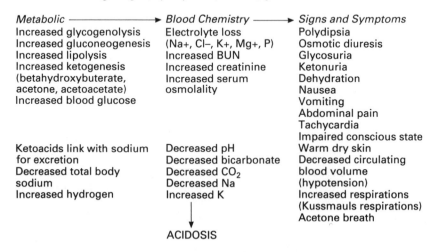

PRECIPITATING FACTORS

INSULIN DEFICIENCY

Decreased glucose uptake
Increased Counter-regulatory Hormone Response
(glucagon, epinephrine, cortisol, growth hormone)

Metabolic ⟶	*Blood Chemistry* ⟶	*Signs and Symptoms*
Increased glycogenolysis	Electrolyte loss	Polydipsia
Increased gluconeogenesis	(Na+, Cl–, K+, Mg+, P)	Osmotic diuresis
Increased lipolysis	Increased BUN	Glycosuria
Increased ketogenesis	Increased creatinine	Ketonuria
(betahydroxybuterate,	Increased serum	Dehydration
acetone, acetoacetate)	osmolality	Nausea
Increased blood glucose		Vomiting
		Abdominal pain
		Tachycardia
		Impaired conscious state
Ketoacids link with sodium	Decreased pH	Warm dry skin
for excretion	Decreased bicarbonate	Decreased circulating
Decreased total body	Decreased CO_2	blood volume
sodium	Decreased Na	(hypotension)
Increased hydrogen	Increased K	Increased respirations
		(Kussmauls respirations)
		Acetone breath

ACIDOSIS

Late signs: coma, absence of Kussmauls respirations, death

Fig. 10.1   An outline of the physiology, signs and symptoms and biochemical changes occurring in the development of diabetes ketoacidosis (DKA).

10.3.2   Aims of treatment of DKA

Treatment aims to:

(1) Correct:
  ● dehydration
  ● electrolyte imbalance
  ● ketoacidosis
  ● hyperglycaemia (to slowly decrease blood glucose to 7–10 mmol/l).
(2) Reverse shock.
(3) Ascertain the cause of DKA and treat appropriately.
(4) Prevent complications of treatment (see section 10.3.6).
(5) Educate/re-educate the patient.

Treatment priorities for the management of DKA are shown in Fig. 10.2.

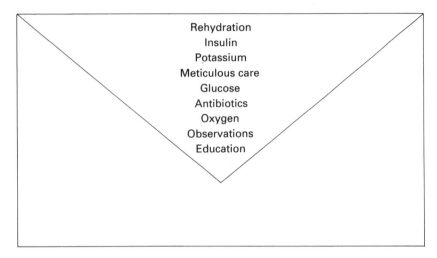

Fig. 10.2 Priorities of management of diabetic ketoacidosis (DKA). (Adapted with permission from Kitalschi, A.E., Matteri, R. & Murphy, M.B. (1982) *Diabetes Care*, 5, 78–87.

10.3.3 Objectives of nursing care

To support the medical team to:

(1) Restore normal hydration, euglycaemia and metabolism.
(2) Prevent complications of DKA including complications occurring as a result of management.
(3) Pay meticulous attention to detail.
(4) Document progress of recovery.
(5) Re-educate/educate the patient about the management of illness at home or general diabetes education if a new diagnosis. Patient education about managing diabetes during illness can be found in Chapter 18.
(6) Ensure follow-up care after discharge, in particular: review of diabetes knowledge, nutritional assessment and physical assessment.

10.3.4 Preparation of the unit to receive the patient

Assemble:

(1) Oxygen and suction (tested to ensure they are in working order).
(2) Intravenous trolley (IV) containing:
   ● dressing tray and antiseptic solution
   ● local anaesthetic
   ● selection of intravenous cannulae

- IV fluids – normal saline, SPPS
- giving sets, burette
- IMED pump or syringe pump
- clear short-acting insulin

Short-acting insulin has a rapid onset of action and quickly promotes transport of glucose into the cells. Intravenous administration is preferred because absorption is more predictable than by the subcutaneous route.

- blood gas syringe
- blood culture bottles.
(3) Cot sides and IV pole.
(4) Blood glucose testing equipment (cleaned, calibrated).
(5) Urine testing equipment:
- Ketodiastix
- Multistix.
(6) Appropriate charts:
- fluid balance
- diabetic record
- conscious state.
(7) Urinary catheterization equipment.
(8) Nasogastric tubes are not usually required.

If the patient is admitted to the intensive care unit, central venous pressures, continuous blood gas and electrocardiogram monitoring may be performed.

10.3.5   Nursing care/observations

The nursing management of DKA involves traditional nursing actions as well as monitoring of the responses to medical therapy.

Initial patient care
Initial patient care is often given in the intensive care unit. The procedure is:

- Maintain the airway.
- Nurse the patient on their side, even if the patient is conscious.
- Gastric stasis and inhalation of vomitus are possible and preventable complications of DKA.
- Ensure strict aseptic technique.

Nursing observations (1–2 hourly)
(1) Observe 'nil orally'. Provide pressure care especially in the elderly patient. Provide mouth care.

(2) Administer IV fluid according to the treatment sheet.

(3) Administer insulin according to the treatment sheet; it is usually given via an insulin infusion adjusted according to blood glucose tests (see section 7.12). (In some cases short-acting insulin may be given intramuscularly.)

(4) Estimate blood glucose levels and confirm biochemically if possible.

(5) Observe strict fluid balance. Record second hourly subtotals of input/ output *from admission*. Urine output should be >30 ml per hour measured in a calibrated collecting device hourly. Report a urine output of <30 ml per hour. Measure specific gravity (SG).

- *Heavy* glycosuria invalidates SG readings.
- Test for ketones.
- Record vomitus.

(6) Monitor central venous pressure.

(7) Monitor conscious state.

(8) Record pulse, respiration and blood pressure.

(9) Administer oxygen via face mask or nasal catheter.

(10) Monitor and report all laboratory results (electrolytes and blood gases).

(11) Report any deterioration of condition immediately.

(12) Physiotherapy may be helpful to prevent pneumonia and emboli due to venous stasis, and to provide passive mobilization.

(13) Administer other drugs as ordered (potassium, calciparine, antibiotics).

(14) Reposition and provide skin care to avoid pressure areas and/or venous stasis.

Subsequent care

As the patient's condition improves:

- Review the frequency of blood glucose testing, decreasing to 4 hourly including the night time
- Allow a light diet and ensure the patient is eating before the IV is removed.
- Administer subcutaneous insulin before the IV is removed.
- Continue to monitor temperature, pulse and respiration every 4 hours.
- Provide support and comfort for the patient.
- Establish the duration of deteriorating control and identify any precipitating factor such as infection.

Plan for:

- Medical follow-up appointment after discharge.
- Nutrition review.

- Education/re-education about appropriate management (for days when the patient is unwell); see Chapter 18.
- Review of medication dosage, especially insulin.

Note: psychiatric consultation should be considered if a patient repeatedly presents in DKA:

- It may be a cry for help/attention.
- Some people, especially adolescent girls, decrease their insulin dose and run blood glucose levels high to control weight.
- Consider sexual assault.

10.3.6   Complications which can occur as a result of DKA

Most complications of DKA are due to complications of treatment and most are avoidable:

(1) Inhalation of vomitus – aspiration pneumonia.
(2) Hypoglycaemia.
(3) Hypokalaemia which may lead to cardiac arrhythmias.
(4) Cerebral oedema.
(5) Myocardial infarction.
(6) Deep venous thrombosis.
(7) Adult respiratory distress syndrome.

Be extra vigilant with:

(1) Elderly patients, especially those with established vascular and coronary disease. Risks include myocardial infarction and deep venous thrombosis.
(2) Children are at increased risk of cerebral oedema, which has a high mortality rate in this group of patients.

10.4   Hyperosmolar non-ketotic coma (HONK)

Hyperosmolar non-ketotic coma is a metabolic disturbance characterized by a marked increase in serum osmolality, the absence of ketones, hyperglycaemia (usually >40 mmol/l) and extreme dehydration. It occurs in people with Type 2 diabetes, but also in people with no previous diagnosis of diabetes.

People with Type 2 diabetes usually still have sufficient endogenous insulin production to prevent the formation of ketones.

HONK predominantly occurs in older people and the onset is associated with severe stress such as infection, extensive burns, myocardial infarction or decreased fluid intake. Other precipitating factors include:

● Some medications: thiazide diuretics, steroids, immunosuppressants.
● Peritoneal dialysis.
● Parenteral nutrition.

There is a high mortality rate associated with HONK.

The nursing care and objectives are similar to those for DKA, but extra vigilance is needed because of the age of these patients. Monitor closely:

● Record strict fluid balance.
● IV fluid rate.
● Blood glucose.
● ECG.
● Urine output.
● Neurological observations.
● Skin integrity.

Observe for deep venous thrombosis or embolism. Subsequent care is as for DKA.

Education may be more difficult because of the age of these patients. It may be difficult to assess the mental state of the patient because of the dehydration. Ensuring that the family/caregivers understand how to care for the patient is important.

Figure 10.3 is an outline of the factors involved in the development of hyperosmolar coma. There are similarities with DKA, with some important differences. Ketone production is absent or minimal, because the patient is usually producing enough endogenous insulin to allow for the ketone bodies to be metabolized and utilized. The degree of dehydration is often greater in HONK and the serum and urine osmolality is increased.

Glass thermometers should not be placed in the mouth if the conscious state is impaired. They can be bitten and break, causing local trauma.

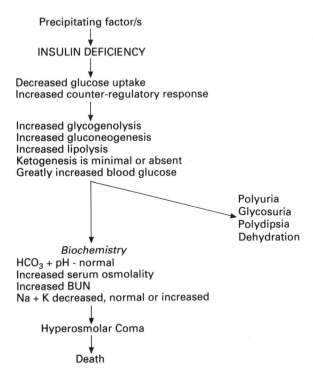

Precipitating factor/s

INSULIN DEFICIENCY

Decreased glucose uptake
Increased counter-regulatory response

Increased glycogenolysis
Increased gluconeogenesis
Increased lipolysis
Ketogenesis is minimal or absent
Greatly increased blood glucose

Polyuria
Glycosuria
Polydipsia
Dehydration

Biochemistry
HCO_3 + pH - normal
Increased serum osmolality
Increased BUN
Na + K decreased, normal or increased

Hyperosmolar Coma

Death

Fig. 10.3   An outline of the development of hyperosmolar coma.

10.5   Further reading

Guyton, A.C. (1966) *Textbook of Medical Physiology*, 7th edn, pp. 806–17. W.B. Saunders, Philadelphia.

Metheny, N.M. (1992) *Fluid Electrolyte Balance*, Chapter 21. Lippincott, Philadelphia.

Sabo, C.E. (1989) Diabetic ketoacidosis, nursing diagnosis and nursing interventions. *Focus on Critical Care*, 16, 21–8.

Walker, M., Marshall, S.M. & Alberti, K.G.M.M. (1989) Clinical aspects of diabetic ketoacidosis. *Diabetes/Metabolism Reviews*, 5, 651–63.

Chapter 11
Care of the Diabetic Person with Cardiac Disease

11.1 Key points

- Chest pain may be atypical in diabetics.
- Watch for weakness, fatigue, increased blood glucose, congestive cardiac failure (CCF).
- Control pain and vomiting.
- Monitor blood glucose.
- Prevent excursions in blood glucose.
- Maintain accurate fluid balance.
- Counsel about risk factors.
- Offer support.

Cardiac disease is a common complication of diabetes, and carries a higher mortality rate than for non-diabetics. There is an association between increasing age, duration of diabetes, the presence of other complications and mortality. Atherosclerosis is more frequent and more severe in diabetics. It occurs at a lower age than in non-diabetics and is more prevalent in women.

Myocardial infarction is 'silent' in 32% of diabetics, which leads to delay in seeking medical attention and may be a factor in the increased mortality rate. The atypical nature of the chest pain may make it difficult for people to accept that they have had a heart attack. Risk factor modification may not be seen as essential. The person may present with hypertension, heart failure, cardiogenic shock or, in the elderly, diabetic ketoacidosis or hyperosmolar coma.

'Silent' infarct means that the classic pain across the chest, down the arm and into the jaw is absent. Only mild discomfort, often mistaken for heartburn, may be present.

Diabetes may be diagnosed at the time of an infarct or during cardiac surgery. Emotional stress, and the associated catecholamine response, leads to increased blood glucose levels in 5% of patients admitted to coronary care units (CCUs). The blood glucose may normalize during convalescence, however counselling about diabetes and its management is important. Tact and sympathy are necessary when informing the patient about the diagnosis of diabetes in these situations.

Patients will usually be cared for in CCUs, but patients in other wards may develop cardiac problems. A longer stay in CCU may be indicated for people with diabetes, because 35% of patients die, often in the second week after the infarct.

11.2   Objectives of care

Nursing care should be planned to avoid constant disturbance of the patient and allow adequate rest and sleep. The objectives of care are to:

- Treat the acute attack according to medical orders and standard protocols.
- Stabilize cardiac status and relieve symptoms.
- Prevent extension of the cardiac abnormality and limit further episodes.
- Retain independence as far as possible.
- Achieve and maintain euglycaemia.
- Provide psychological support.
- Prevent complications while in hospital.
- Counsel about risk factor modification.
- Educate/re-educate about diabetes.

11.3   Nursing responsibilities

(1) To provide psychological, educational and physical care.
(2) To monitor blood glucose, 2–4 hourly depending on stability and route of insulin administration.
(3) To provide adequate pain relief, and to control vomiting, which can exacerbate high blood glucose levels.
(4) To perform treatment according to the medical orders for the specific cardiac abnormality.
(5) To administer insulin:
   - Many patients on OHAs are changed to insulin during the acute phase to improve blood glucose control.
   - Insulin is usually administered via an infusion at least for the first 48 hours. Only clear insulin is used. Insulin infusions are discussed in Chapter 7. The patient should be eating and drinking normally before the infusion is removed, and a dose of subcutaneous insulin given to prevent hyperglycaemia developing.
(6) Medications: OHAs should be stopped while the patient is having

insulin to reduce the risk of hypoglycaemia and lactic acidosis. Thiazide diuretics can:

● Increase blood glucose levels.

● Cause hypokalaemia.

Non-cardiac-specific beta-blocking agents may mask the signs of hypoglycaemia. Patients who are normally tablet controlled will require support and education about the use of insulin. It should be explained that insulin is being given to increase the glucose available to the myocardium and decrease free fatty acids in the blood. Most patients can be controlled by oral agents when the acute crisis has resolved.

(7) Physical status:

● Monitor fluid balance and maintain accurate charts, to help assess kidney function.

● Monitor blood pressure, lying and standing. Some antihypertensive medications can cause orthostatic hypotension. Counsel the patient to change position gradually, especially on getting out of bed or out of a chair.

● Monitor ECG.

● Observe for weakness, fatigue, CCF or unexplained hyperglycaemia which may indicate a further infarct.

● Provide appropriate skin care to prevent dryness and pressure areas.

(8) Blood tests:

● Monitor serum electrolytes, cardiac enzymes, blood gases and potassium levels. Report abnormalities to the doctor promptly. Fluctuating potassium levels can cause or exacerbate cardiac arrhythmias.

● Prevent hypoglycaemia by careful monitoring of blood glucose and carbohydrate intake.

The patient may not recognize the signs of hypoglycaemia if:

● Autonomic neuropathy is present.

● Non-selective beta blocking agents are used.

Neuroglycopenic signs of hypoglycaemia (confusion, slurred speech or behaviour change) may predominate.

11.4   Medical tests/procedures (see Chapter 13)

(1) The eyes should be assessed *before* thrombolytic medications are commenced. If proliferative retinopathy is present, bleeding into the back of the eye may occur, requiring urgent treatment.

(2) Diagnostic procedures which require the use of contrast dyes, e.g. angiograms, have been associated with renal complications.
Ensure adequate hydration before and after procedures and monitor urine output, especially in elderly people or those with renal disease.

11.5   Rehabilitation

(1) Encourage activity within tolerance limits. Refer for physiotherapy/occupational therapy.
(2) Encourage independence.
(3) Counsel about resumption of normal activity, including sexual intercourse, after discharge home.
(4) Ensure diabetic education/re-education is available. Refer to diabetes educator, dietitian and physiotherapist. Education should also address the risk factors involved in the development of cardiac disease (see section 11.6). Particular areas of concern are:
  - Recognition of hypoglycaemia.
  - Correct insulin technique.
  - Correct blood glucose monitoring technique.
  - Possible indicators of further cardiac problems.
  - Dietary assessment and advice.
  - Risk factor modification.

11.6   Modification of risk factors associated with the development of cardiac disease

The patient requires both information and support to motivate him to:

  - Stop smoking.
  - Avoid high calorie foods and high fat intake to achieve sensible weight reduction.
  - Increase regular exercise/activities.
  - Achieve acceptable blood glucose levels.

11.7   Further reading

Gotch, P. (1986) Atherosclerosis as a complication of diabetes. *Focus on Critical Care*, 13, 9–15.
Jowett, N. (1986) Diabetic heart disease. *Nursing Times*, 29 October, 33–4.
Webster, R. & Thompson, R. (1991) The diabetic patient in the coronary care unit: a nursing perspective. *Practical Diabetes*, 8, 13–17.

Chapter 12
Management During Surgical Procedures

12.1 Key points

- Assess pre-operatively.
- Morning procedure if possible.
- Never omit insulin in Type 1 patients.
- Stabilize diabetes before procedure.
- Cease oral agents 24–36 hours pre-operatively.
- Watch for hypo/hyperglycaemia.
- Instruct patient carefully.

12.2 Introduction

People with diabetes undergo surgery for the same reasons as those without diabetes, however because of the long-term complications of diabetes they are more likely to require:

- Cardiac procedures.
- Angioplasty.
- Bypass surgery.
- Amputations (toes, feet).
- Eye surgery (cataracts, retinal detachment, carpal tunnel decompression).

Surgery results in endocrine, metabolic and long-term effects which have implications for the management of people with diabetes undergoing surgery. These effects are summarized in Table 12.1. These factors must be controlled in order to promote healing and reduce the risk of infection post-operatively. Fasting causes an increase in the catabolic hormones, and can lead to electrolyte imbalances and hyperglycaemia in diabetics, especially given that the insulin response is impaired or absent in diabetics.

Table 12.1 Hormonal, metabolic and long-term effects of surgery.

Hormonal	Metabolic	Long-term effects
↑ secretion of epinephrine, norepinephrine, ACTH, cortisol and growth hormone ↓ secretion of insulin Insulin resistance	Hyperglycaemia ↓ glucose utilization ↑ gluconeogenesis ↑ protein catabolism ↑ lipolysis with ↑ production of free fatty acids and ketone bodies ↑ risk of cerebrovascular accident, myocardial infarction Electrolyte disorders ↑metabolic rate ↓ blood pressure	Loss of lean body mass – impaired wound healing, resistance to infection Loss of adipose tissue Deficiency of essential amino acids, vitamins, minerals, and essential fatty acids

12.3 Aims of management

(1) To achieve normal metabolism by supplying sufficient insulin to counterbalance the increase in stress hormones during fasting and surgery (blood glucose between 5 and 10 mmol/l).
(2) To achieve this with regimes which minimize the possibility of errors.
(3) To ensure that the patient undergoes surgery in the best possible physical condition.
(4) To prevent:
   ● hypoglycaemia
   ● complications of surgery
   ● electrolyte imbalance
   ● worsening of pre-existing diabetic complications
   ● infection.
(5) To avoid undue psychological stress.

12.4 Pre-operative nursing care

Good pre-operative nursing care is important for both major and minor procedures. The patient may be admitted 2 to 3 days before the operation to stabilize glucose levels. If possible, schedule for a morning procedure.

12.4.1 Nursing actions

(1) Confirm time of operation.

(2) Explain procedure and post-operative care to patient. Those patients controlled by OHAs or by diet may require insulin *during surgery and immediately post-operatively*. They should be aware of this possibility. Insulin during the operative period does not mean that diet- or tablet-controlled patients will remain on insulin when they recover from the procedure.

(3) Ensure all documentation is completed:
- consent form
- medication chart
- monitoring guidelines
- chest X-ray and other X-rays, scans, MRI (magnetic imaging resonance)
- ECG.

(4) Sulphonylureas are usually ceased 24 hours pre-operatively; metformin and chlorpropamide 36 hours pre-operatively. Check medical orders.

(5) Encourage cessation of smoking (in patients who smoke).

(6) Assess:
- metabolic status: blood glucose control, hydration status, nutritional status, presence of anaemia, diabetic symptoms
- educational level and understanding of diabetes
- family support
- any known allergies or drug reactions
- presence of diabetic complications (renal, hepatic, cardiac, presence of neuropathy)
- patients with autonomic neuropathy pose special problems while under the anaesthetic: gastroparesis delays gastric emptying and the stomach can be full despite fasting, increasing the possibility of regurgitation and inhalation of vomitus; or the vasoconstrictive response to reduced cardiac output may be absent
- current medications
- presence of infection; check feet.

Note: complications should be managed before operation where possible.

12.4.2 Day of operation

Pre-medication and routine preparation for the scheduled operative procedure should be performed according to the treatment sheet and standard protocols.

Morning procedure

(1) Ensure oral medications have been ceased.

(2) Fast from 12 midnight.

(3) Ascertain insulin regime: commence insulin infusion (see Chapter 7).

(4) Monitor blood glucose 2 hourly.

Afternoon procedure

(1) Fast after an early light breakfast.

(2) Ensure oral medications have been ceased.

(3) Ascertain insulin dose, usually $\frac{1}{2}$ to $\frac{1}{3}$ of usual dose (best given after an IV has been commenced).

(4) It is preferable for IV therapy to be commenced in the ward to:
   - prevent dehydration
   - decrease the risk of hypoglycaemia.

   This will depend on the surgical and anaesthetic team and usual hospital procedure.

(5) Monitor blood glucose.

The anaesthetist is usually responsible for the intra-operative blood glucose monitoring. The patient is dependent on this monitoring to detect hypoglycaemia. The usual signs will be masked by the anaesthetic. Precautions are needed to avoid regurgitation and aspiration, cardiac arrhythmias and postural hypotension in patients with autonomic neuropathy.

12.5 Post-operative nursing responsibilities

12.5.1 Immediate care

(1) Monitor and record vital signs according to instructions.

(2) Maintain an accurate fluid balance.

(3) Monitor blood and urinary glucose/ketones initially 2 hourly.

(4) Observe dressings for signs of haemorrhage or excess discharge.

(5) Ensure drain tubes are patent and draining.

(6) Document all information relating to input and output, especially:

Input	Output
IV Fluid	Drainage from wound
Oral	Vomitus
EN and TPN	Diarrhoea
	Urine

(7) Maintain care of IV insulin infusion.

(8) Ensure vomiting and pain are controlled.

(9) Ensure psychological needs are addressed, e.g. body image change.

(10) Ensure referral to appropriate allied health professional, e.g. physiotherapist.

12.5.2   Ongoing care

(1) Document all data accurately on the appropriate charts.
(2) Prevent complications:
 ● infection – aseptic dressing technique including IV sites
 ● venous thrombosis – anti-embolic stockings
 ● hypo/hyperglycaemia.
(3) Diabetes education.
(4) Rehabilitation.

Antibiotics and heparin should be administered according to individual patient requirements and medical orders.

Note: insulin therapy is continued for tablet-controlled patients until they are eating a normal diet and blood glucose levels are stabilized.

12.6   Minor procedures

Minor surgery may be performed on an outpatient basis. The metabolic risks described are still a consideration if the patient is expected to fast for the procedure. Ensure that the procedure is fully explained to the patient at the time of making the appointment. Give *written* instructions about insulin, oral agents and other medications. Pre-operative care is the same as for major surgery on the day of operation as regards:

● Oral agents.
● Morning procedure is preferred.

Guidelines for patient instructions
Examples of patient instructions for people undergoing outpatient procedures can be found in Patient Instruction Sheets 2 (a) and (b).

Morning procedure
(1) No insulin in the morning on the day of the procedure.
(2) Test blood glucose before coming to hospital.
(3) Fast from 12 midnight.
(4) Bring insulin to hospital.
(5) Advise patient to have someone available to drive them home after the procedure.

Afternoon procedure
(1) Light breakfast (e.g. tea and toast).
(2) Fast after this breakfast.
(3) Test blood glucose before coming to hospital.
(4) Give insulin dose according to blood glucose test as ordered by the doctor.
(5) Explain before discharge:
  ● the risk of hypoglycaemia if not eating
  ● what to take for pain relief
  ● when to recommence OHAs/insulin
  ● what and when to eat.

In both cases
(1) Test blood glucose at the end of the procedure and before discharge.
(2) Ensure the patient has appropriate doctor's appointments.
(3) Ensure the patient has someone to accompany him/her home.
(4) Allay concerns about the procedure.
(5) Provide appropriate care according to the medical orders.
(6) Inspect all wounds before discharge.
(7) It is not advisable to drive, operate machinery or drink alcohol until the following day.

Ensure patient understands meaning of 'fast'.

12.7 Emergency procedures

The specific management will depend on the nature of the emergency. If possible the metabolic status should be stabilized before surgery is commenced. The minimum requirements are:

(1) Adequate hydration.
(2) Freedom from hyperglycaemia and especially ketoacidosis (DKA). If the patient presents with an abdominal emergency ensure that it is not due to DKA before operating.
  Specific treatment depends on:

● The nature of the emergency
● The time of the last food intake
● The time and type of the last insulin dose
● Blood glucose levels.

12.8   Further reading

Alberti, K.C.G.M., Gill, G.V. & Elliott, M.J. (1982) Insulin delivery during surgery in the diabetic patient. *Diabetes Care*, 5, (Suppl. 1). 65–77.

PATIENT INSTRUCTION SHEET 2:
(A) EXAMPLE INSTRUCTIONS FOR DIABETIC
PATIENTS ON ORAL HYPOGLYCAEMIC AGENTS
HAVING PROCEDURES AS OUTPATIENTS
UNDER SEDATION OR GENERAL ANAESTHESIA.

EXAMPLE INSTRUCTIONS FOR DIABETIC PATIENTS ON ORAL HYPOGLYCAEMIC AGENTS HAVING PROCEDURES AS OUTPATIENTS UNDER SEDATION OR GENERAL ANAESTHESIA

Patient's Name: .... UR: ....

Time & Date of Appointment: ....

**IT IS IMPORTANT THAT YOU INFORM NURSING STAFF
THAT YOU HAVE DIABETES**

Morning

If your diabetes is controlled by diet and/or diabetic tablets and you are going to the operating theatre in the morning:

- take nothing by mouth from midnight
- test your blood glucose
- omit your morning diabetic tablets.

Afternoon

If your diabetes is controlled by diet and/or diabetic tablets and you are going to the operating theatre in the afternoon:

- have a light breakfast only (coffee/tea, 2 slices of toast with spread), and nothing by mouth thereafter
- test your blood glucose
- omit your morning diabetic tablets.

Delete the inappropriate paragraph

If you have any questions:

Contact: .... Telephone: ....

PATIENT INSTRUCTION SHEET 2:
(B) EXAMPLE INSTRUCTIONS FOR DIABETIC PATIENTS ON INSULIN HAVING PROCEDURES AS OUTPATIENTS UNDER SEDATION OR GENERAL ANAESTHESIA.

EXAMPLE OF INSTRUCTIONS FOR DIABETIC PATIENTS

ON INSULIN HAVING PROCEDURES AS OUTPATIENTS

UNDER SEDATION OR GENERAL ANAESTHESIA

Patient's Name: .... UR: ....

Time & Date of Appointment: ....

**IT IS IMPORTANT THAT YOU INFORM NURSING STAFF
THAT YOU HAVE DIABETES**

Morning

If your diabetes is controlled by insulin and you are going to the operating theatre in the morning:

- take nothing by mouth from midnight

- test your blood glucose

- omit your morning insulin.

Afternoon

If your diabetes is controlled by insulin and you are going to the operating theatre in the afternoon:

- have a light breakfast only (coffee/tea, 2 slices of toast with spread), and nothing by mouth thereafter

- test your blood glucose

- take .... units of insulin.

Delete the inappropriate paragraph

If you have any questions:

Contact: .... Telephone: ....

Chapter 13
Care During Medical Tests and Procedures

13.1 Key points

- Careful preparation.
- Monitor blood glucose regularly.
- Monitor fluid balance.
- Never omit insulin in Type 1 diabetes.
- Radio-opaque dyes may cause tubular necrosis in the elderly diabetic; monitor fluid balance.

Management protocols for patients undergoing medical tests/procedures such as X-rays, gastroscopy or laser therapy are not as intricate as those for ketoacidosis or major surgery. However, vigilant nursing care is equally as important to prevent excursions in blood glucose levels and psychological stress.

13.2 The objectives of care

(1) As for surgical procedures, Chapter 12.
(2) To ensure correct preparation for the test.
(3) To ensure the procedure has been explained to the patient.
(4) To provide written instructions for the patient if the test is to be performed on an outpatient basis.

13.3 General nursing management requirements

(1) Insulin/oral hypoglycaemic agents:
   - insulin is *never omitted* in Type 1 diabetics
   - if the patient needs to fast, insulin should be adjusted accordingly
   - OHAs are usually withheld on the morning of the test
   - ensure written medical instructions are available, including for after the procedure.
(2) Aim for a morning procedure if fasting is required.

(3) Monitor blood glucose before and after the test and during the night (3 AM) if fasting and in hospital.

(4) Observe for signs of dehydration. Maintain fluid balance chart if:
- fasting is prolonged
- bowel preparations are required (some may lead to a fluid deficit)
- an IV infusion is commenced
- dehydration in elderly people may predispose them to kidney damage if a radio-opaque contrast medium is used.

An IV infusion may dilute some radio-opaque dyes. The advice of the radiographer should be sought if IV therapy is necessary. Continue IV infusions after the procedure to wash out dyes and contrast medium.

(5) Control nausea and vomiting and pain which can increase the blood glucose level.

(6) Ensure the patient can eat and drink normally after the procedure to avoid hypoglycaemia.

(7) Assess puncture sites (e.g. angiography) before discharge.

(8) Recommence medications as per the medical order.

13.4 Eye procedures

People with diabetes are more prone to visual impairment and blindness than the general population. The eye manifestations of diabetes can affect all ocular structures. The time of appearance, rate of progression and severity of eye disease vary between individuals. However almost all patients have some evidence of damage after 25 years of diabetes.

Retinopathy (a common problem occurring in diabetes) is symptomless and may remain undetected if the eyes are not examined regularly by an ophthalmologist. Fluorescein angiography and retinal photography may aid in determining the severity of the disease. Management aims at conserving vision, and laser therapy is often effective in this respect.

13.4.1 Care of patient having fluorescein angiography

Fluorescein angiography is usually an outpatient procedure. The reasons for the test and the procedure should be carefully explained to the patient. They should be aware that:

- Transient nausea may occur.
- The skin and urine may become yellow for 12–24 hours.
- Drinking adequate amounts of fluid will help flush the dye out of the system.

13.4.2   Care of the patient having laser therapy (photocoagulation)

'Laser' is an acronym for light amplification stimulated emission of radiation. There are many types of lasers. The ones that are used to treat diabetic patients are the argon, krypton and diode lasers. The lasers absorb light, which is converted to heat, which coagulates the tissue. Laser therapy is frequently used to treat diabetic retinopathy and glaucoma.

Goals of photocoagulation
To maintain vision:

- By allowing fluid exchange to occur, reducing fluid accumulation in the retina.
- To photocoagulate the retina, which is ischaemic, and thereby cause new vessels (which may haemorrhage) to regress.

Laser therapy is usually performed on an outpatient basis. Fasting is not required and medication adjustment is unnecessary.

Laser therapy may not increase vision, but can prevent further loss of vision.

Nursing responsibilities
Ensure the purpose of laser therapy has been explained to the patient. The patient should know that:

(1) Before the procedure:
- the pupil of the eye will be dilated
- anaesthetic drops may be used
- the laser beam causes bright lights
- vision will be blurred for some time after the laser treatment
- they should test their blood glucose before and after laser treatment
- they should not drive home.
(2) After the procedure:
- sunglasses will protect the eye and help reduce discomfort
- spots may be seen for 24–48 hours
- there may be some discomfort for 2–3 weeks
- headache may develop after the procedure
- paracetamol may be taken to relieve pain

Aspirin is best avoided because of its anticoagulant effect. If new vessels are present due to retinopathy they may bleed, threatening sight.

- activities which will increase intraocular pressure for 24–36 hours, e.g. lifting heavy objects, straining at stool, should be avoided

- night vision may be temporarily decreased
- vision to the side may be permanently diminished; this is known as 'tunnel vision'.

Blurred vision does not necessarily indicate serious eye disease. It can occur during both hypo- and hyperglycaemia. Vision may also become worse when diabetic control is improved, e.g. after commencement of insulin therapy. Although this is distressing for the patient, vision usually improves in 6–8 weeks. Prescriptions for glasses obtained in these circumstances may be inappropriate. Glasses are best obtained when the eyes settle down.

The nursing care of people who are vision impaired is discussed in Chapter 14.

13.4.3   Care of the patient having radiocontrast media injected

Radiocontrast media are excreted through the kidneys. Fasting is often required. The patient can become dehydrated, especially if kept waiting for long periods, and kidney complications can occur. Patients most at risk:

- Are over 50 years old.
- Have established kidney disease.
- Have had diabetes for more than 10 years.
- Are hypertensive.
- Have proteinuria.
- Have an elevated serum creatinine.

Kidney problems caused by radiocontrast media may not produce symptoms. A decreased urine output following procedures requiring radiocontrast media may indicate kidney damage.

Management
(1) Ensure appropriate preparation has been carried out.
(2) Ensure the patient is well hydrated before the procedure (intravenous therapy may be needed).
(3) Maintain an accurate fluid balance chart.
(4) Avoid delays in performing the procedure.
(5) Monitor urine output after the procedure.
(6) Assess serum creatinine after the procedure.
(7) Good diabetic control.
(8) Encourage the patient to drink to help flush out the contrast media.

Chapter 14
Special Circumstances

This chapter briefly outlines the management and nursing responsibilities associated with the care of diabetic patients receiving enteral and total parenteral nutrition (TPN), continuous ambulatory peritoneal dialysis (CAPD), those with cancer as an added disease process, and those with significant loss of vision.

These conditions are often cared for in specialized units by specialist nursing staff. In some cases the patient is responsible for caring for their own TPN or CAPD at home. Therefore, it is important for the general nurse (especially domiciliary nurses) to have a knowledge of the nursing care required.

The policies and procedures of the employing institution for the care of central lines, dialysis equipment and nasogastric tubes should be adhered to.

Enteral and parenteral nutrition

14.1 Key points

- Strict asepsis.
- Ensure patency of tubes.
- Weigh regularly.
- Maintain accurate fluid balance chart.
- Monitor blood glucose.
- Monitor serum electrolytes, albumin and urea.

Enteral and parenteral nutrition supply nutritional requirements in special circumstances. Often the patient is extremely ill or has undergone major gastrointestinal, head or neck surgery or has gastroparesis diabeticorum, a rare complication specific to diabetes.

14.2 Aims of therapy

(1) Decrease anxiety associated with the procedure by thorough explanation.
(2) Prevent sepsis.
(3) Maintain an acceptable blood glucose range (4–10 mmol/l).
(4) Maintain normal urea, electrolytes, LFTs and blood gas levels.
(5) Supply adequate nutrition in terms of protein, fat and carbohydrate.
(6) Achieve positive nitrogen balance.
(7) Prevent complications of therapy.
(8) The long-term aim of enteral/parenteral feeding is the return of the patient to oral feeding.

14.3 Routes of administration

14.3.1 Enteral

This route supplies nutrients and fluids via an enteral tube when the oral route is inadequate or obstructed. Feeds are administered via a nasogastric, duodenal, jejunal or gastrostomy tube.

Mode of administration
(1) Bolus instillation: may result in distension and delayed gastric emptying. Aspiration may occur. Diarrhoea may be a complication. *This method is not suitable for diabetics who have autonomic neuropathy, especially gastroparesis.*

(2) Continuous infusion: via gravity infusion or pump. May lead to hyperinsulinaemia.

The strength of the feeds should be increased gradually to prevent a sudden overwhelming glucose load in the bloodstream. An IV insulin infusion may be needed to control blood glucose levels.

The feeds usually contain protein, fat and carbohydrate. The carbohydrate is in the form of dextrose, either 25% or 40%, and extra insulin may be needed to control the blood glucose. A balance must be achieved between caloric requirements and blood glucose levels. Patients who are controlled by OHAs will usually need insulin while on enteral feeding.

14.3.2   Parenteral

This is administration of nutrients and fluids by routes other than the alimentary canal: intravenously via a peripheral or central line.

Mode of administration
Parenteral supplements may be partial or total.

(1) Peripheral: used after gastrointestinal surgery and in malabsorption states. Peripheral access is usually reserved for people in whom central access is difficult or sometimes as a supplement to oral/enteral feeds. Not suitable if a high dextrose supplement is needed because dextrose irritates the veins, causing considerable discomfort.
(2) Central: supplies maximum nutrition in the form of protein, carbohydrate, fats, trace elements, vitamins and electrolytes. For example, in patients with cancer or burns, larger volumes can be given than via the peripheral route. Provides long-term access: silastic catheters can be left *in situ* indefinitely. If patients are at risk of sepsis, the site of the central line is rotated weekly using strict aseptic technique. Insulin may be added to the bag (*clear* insulin only); the use of a central line allows the patient to remain mobile, which aids digestion.

14.4   Choice of formula

The particular formula selected depends on the nutritional assessment and absorptive capacity of the patient. It is usual to begin with half strength formula and gradually increase to full strength as tolerated. The aim is to supply adequate:

● Fluid.
● Protein.
● Carbohydrate.

● Vitamins and minerals.
● Sodium spread evenly over the 24 hours.

Nutritional requirements may vary from week to week; careful monitoring of the patient and formula adjustment are essential.

14.5 Nursing responsibilities

14.5.1 Care of nasogastric tube

(1) Explain purpose of tube to patient.
(2) Check position of the tube regularly.
(3) Confirm position with X-ray.
(4) Change position in nose daily to avoid pressure areas.
(5) Flush regularly to ensure patency.
(6) Check residual gastric volumes regularly to avoid gastric distension and the possibility of aspiration.

14.5.2 Care of IV and central lines

(1) Dress regularly.
(2) Check position of central line on chest X-ray.
(3) Maintain strict aseptic technique.
(4) Maintain patency, usually by intermittent installation of heparinized saline (weekly or when line is changed).
(5) Patients should be supine when the central catheter is disconnected and IV giving sets should be carefully primed to minimize the risk of air embolism.
(6) Check catheter for signs of occlusion (e.g. resistance to infusion or difficulty in withdrawing blood sample). Reposition patient; if occlusion still present consult doctor.
(7) Observe exit site for any tenderness, redness, swelling. If bleeding occurs around suture or exit apply pressure and notify doctor.

14.5.3 General nursing care

(1) Maintain an accurate fluid balance chart, including loss from stomas, drain tubes, vomitus and diarrhoea.
(2) Monitor serum albumin, urea and electrolytes to determine nutritional requirements.
(3) Ensure dietitian referral.
(4) Weigh regularly (weekly) at the same time, using same scales and wearing similar clothing.

(5) Monitor blood glucose regularly, at least 4 hourly, initially. If elevated, be aware of possibility of a hyperosmolar event (see Chapter 10). If stable, monitor urine QID and test blood glucose if glycosuria occurs.
(6) Record temperature, pulse and respiration and report if elevated (>38°C) or if any respiratory distress occurs.
(7) Check the date and appearance of all infusions before administration.
(8) Medications are given separately to the formula except insulin and anticoagulants, which may be added to the formula. Follow pump instructions carefully.
(9) Measure skin fold thickness and mid-arm muscle circumference to ascertain weight loss/gain.

14.5.4 Care when recommencing oral feeds

(1) Monitor blood glucose very carefully. Long-acting insulin is usually commenced so there is a risk of hypoglycaemia.
(2) Monitor any nausea or vomiting, describe vomitus.
(3) Maintain accurate fluid balance chart, usually 2 hourly subtotals.

Dialysis and continuous ambulatory peritoneal dialysis

14.6 Key points

- Careful assessment of diabetic and uraemic status.
- Education about dialysis and diabetes.
- Monitor blood glucose.
- Aseptic technique.
- Ensure patency of tubes.
- Use only short-acting insulin in diasylate bags.

14.7 Introduction

Kidney damage is thought to develop in up to 50% of Type 1 diabetics. The incidence has possibly been under-rated in Type 2 diabetics, and is now thought to approach that of Type 1. Renal failure, often fatal, occurs in 25% of patients diagnosed with diabetes before age 30. Malaise and lethargy may also be attributable to decreased renal function in some patients.

The development of renal problems is insidious and frank proteinuria may not be present for 7 to 10 years after the onset of renal disease. Microalbuminuria, on the other hand, is detectable up to 5 years before protein is found in the urine. Regular urine collections to measure micro-albumin, early treatment of blood pressure (even mild elevations) and good metabolic control can help preserve kidney function. Diabetic kidney disease is often accompanied by retinopathy, especially in Type 1 patients.

Patients with significant renal disease on OHAs are usually changed to insulin therapy. Insulin requirements often decrease. Insulin and many OHAs are degraded in the kidney. Kidney damage may delay their degradation, increasing the risk of hypoglycaemia.

14.8 Renal dialysis

Dialysis can be used in the management of diabetic kidney disease. Dialysis is a filtering process which removes excess fluid and accumulated waste products from the blood. It may be required on a temporary basis or for extended periods of time. Some patients may eventually receive a kidney transplant.

There are several forms of dialysis in use:

Haemodialysis (artificial kidney)
Blood is pumped through an artificial membrane then returned to the circulation. Good venous access is required and special training in management.

Peritoneal dialysis
The filtering occurs across the peritoneum. This form of dialysis is an excellent method of treating kidney failure, in people without diabetes as well. The uraemia, hypertension and blood glucose can be well controlled without increasing the risk of infection, if aseptic techniques are adhered to.

Continuous ambulatory peritoneal dialysis (CAPD)
CAPD is a form of peritoneal dialysis in which dialysate is continually present in the abdominal cavity. The fluid is drained and replaced three or four times each day. The patient can be managed at home, which has psychological advantages, once the care of equipment is understood and the patient is metabolically stable.

CAPD can also be used post-operatively to control uraemia related to acute tubular necrosis or early transplant rejection.

14.8.1   Priorities of dialysis treatment

(1) Removal of waste products and excess fluids from the blood (urea and protein).
(2) To provide adequate nutrition and safe serum electrolytes, and to prevent acidosis.
(3) Patient comfort.
(4) To prevent complications of treatment.
(5) To provide information and support to the patient.
(6) To ensure privacy.

14.9   Objectives of care

(1) To assess the patient carefully in relation to:
 ● knowledge of diabetes
 ● preventative health care practices
 ● ability to use aseptic technique
 ● usual diabetic control
 ● presence of other diabetic complications
 ● support available (family, relatives)
 ● motivation for self-care
 ● uraemic state.

(2) To ensure thorough instruction about administration of diasylate and intraperitoneal medication (insulin).

(3) To ensure a regular meal pattern with appropriate carbohydrate in relation to diasylate fluid.

(4) To maintain skin integrity by ensuring technique is aseptic especially in relation to catheter exit site and skin care.

(5) To monitor urea, creatinine and electrolytes carefully.

(6) To provide psychological support.

(7) To encourage simple appropriate exercise.

(8) To ensure adequate dental care and regular dental assessments.

(9) To prevent pain and discomfort, especially associated with the weight of the diasylate.

(10) To ensure the patient reports illness or high temperatures immediately.

14.10 Nursing responsibilities

(1) Meticulous skin care.

(2) Inspect catheter exit site daily, report any redness, swelling, pain or discharge.

(3) Monitor fluid balance carefully:
- weigh all fluid to be instilled
- measure all drainage
- maintain progressive total of input and output
- report a positive balance of more than 1 litre
- report a negative balance as ordered by the doctor.

(4) Monitor blood glucose.

(5) Monitor temperature, pulse and respiration, and report abnormalities.

(6) Monitor nutritional status – intake and biochemistry results.

(7) Weigh daily to monitor fluid intake and nutritional status.

(8) Ensure patency of tubes and monitor colour of outflow. Report if:
- cloudy
- yellow (possible urine contamination)
- faecal contamination
- very little outflow (tube blocked).

(9) Report lethargy and malaise which may be due to uraemia or high blood glucose levels.

(10) Warm diasylate before administration and prior to the addition of prescribed drugs to decrease the possibility of abdominal cramps.

(11) Oral fluid intake may be restricted – provide mouth care and ice to suck.

(12) Assess self-care potential:
- blood glucose testing

- adding medication to bags
- aseptic technique
- psychological ability to cope.

(13) Protect the kidney during routine tests and procedures by avoiding dehydration and infection (Chapter 13).

14.11   Commencing CAPD in patients on insulin

Prior to commencing intraperitoneal insulin, most patients require a 24 hour blood glucose profile to assess the degree of glycaemia in order to calculate insulin requirements accurately. The glucose profile should be carried out following catheter implantation, with the patient stabilized on a CAPD regimen.

14.11.1   Suggested method

(1) Obtain venous access for drawing blood samples.
(2) Obtain hourly blood glucose levels for 24 hours.
(3) At each bag exchange send:
- 10 ml new dianeal fluid for glucose analysis
- 10 ml drained dianeal fluid for glucose and insulin analysis to the appropriate laboratory.

14.12   Protocol for insulin administration in diabetics on CAPD – based on four bag changes each day

(1) Calculate usual daily requirement of insulin and double it.
(2) Divide this amount between the four bags.

Note: the overnight bag should contain half of the daytime dose.

Example

Usual total insulin units	= 60 units
multiply this amount by 2	= 120 units
divide 120 units by 4 exchanges	= 30 units/bag
3 daily exchanges	= 30 units/bag
overnight exchange	= 15 units/bag

Adjustments for the dextrose concentration of the diasylate may be necessary. Intraperitoneal insulin requirements are usually one third higher than the amount needed before CAPD.

14.13 Education of patient about CAPD

The patient should be instructed to:

(1) Not have a shower or bath for the first 6 weeks after the catheter is inserted.
(2) Always carefully wash hands prior to changing the bags.
(3) Wear loose fitting clothes over exit site.
(4) Examine feet daily for signs of bruising, blisters, cuts or swelling.
(5) Wear gloves when gardening or using caustic cleaners.
(6) Avoid water bottles and electric blankets because sensory neuropathy can diminish pain perception and result in burns.
(7) Avoid constrictive stockings or wearing new shoes for a long period of time.
(8) Wash cuts or scratches immediately with soap and water and apply a mild antiseptic (for example betadine ointment). Any wound that does not improve within 24 to 36 hours or shows signs of infection (redness, pain, tenderness) must be reported promptly.
(9) Bag exchanges should be carried out around meal times.
(10) **Only short-acting *clear* insulin must be used in bags**.
(11) Adjust insulin doses according to diet, activity and blood glucose levels and at the physician's discretion.
(12) Accurately monitor blood glucose 4 hourly. A blood glucose meter may be required.
(13) Provide written information.

Immediate help should be sought if any of the following occur:

● Decreased appetite.
● Bad breath/taste in mouth.
● Muscle cramps.
● Generalized itch.
● Nausea and vomiting, especially in the morning.
● Decreased urine output.
● Signs of urinary infection such as burning or scalding.

Diabetes and cancer

14.14   Key points

- Provide psychological support.
- Use aseptic techniques.
- Monitor nutritional status.
- Control pain, nausea, vomiting.
- Monitor blood glucose.

Cancer occurs in people with diabetes with the same frequency as in the general population, with the exception of cancer of the pancreas. However, there is no evidence that diabetes leads to pancreatic cancer.

The management of the cancer itself is the same for people with diabetes as for other people; however some extra considerations apply. Cancer cells trap amino acids for their own use, limiting the protein available for normal functions. Weight loss, increased gluconeogenesis and hypoalbuminaemia occur. For the diabetic this can lead to hyperglycaemia and decreased insulin production, with consequent effects on blood glucose control, and may lead to delayed wound healing.

Diabetic management should be considered in relation to the prognosis and the anti-cancer therapy. Preventing the long-term complications of diabetes may be irrelevant in these people, therefore striving for very good control may not be recommended.

Specific treatment will vary according to the type of cancer the patient has. Diagnosis of some types of cancer (e.g. endocrine tumours) can involve prolonged fasting and radiological imaging and/or other radiological procedures. The appropriate care should be given in these circumstances (see Chapter 13).

Steroid therapy is frequently used in the treatment of cancers, and to relieve cerebral oedema. The steroids may be given over a prolonged time or in large doses for a short period. Steroids are antagonistic to insulin and their use can lead to high blood glucose levels, even in people without diabetes. Therefore urine and blood glucose will be monitored regularly in these patients.

14.15   Objectives of care

(1) To achieve as good a lifestyle as possible for as long as possible.
(2) To achieve an acceptable blood glucose range in order to avoid the distressing symptoms associated with hyperglycaemia.

(3) To prevent malnutrition, dehydration with possible consequent hypoglycaemia, delayed healing and decreased resistance to infection.
(4) To control pain.
(5) To prevent trauma.
(6) To monitor renal and hepatic function during administration of cytotoxic drugs.
(7) To provide education and psychological support.

14.16   Nursing responsibilities

(1) To provide a safe environment.
(2) To consider the psychological aspects of having cancer and diabetes (fear of death, body image changes, denial).
(3) To ensure appropriate diabetic education if diabetes develops as a consequence of the altered metabolism of cancer.
(4) To attend to pressure areas, including the feet and around nasogastric tubes.
(5) To provide oral care, and ensure a dental consultation occurs.
(6) To control nausea, vomiting and pain.
(7) To monitor blood glucose levels.
(8) To chart accurately fluid balance, blood glucose, TPR, weight.
(9) To ensure referral to the dietitian, psychologist, diabetes educator.
(10) To be aware of the possibility of hypoglycaemia if the patient is not eating or is vomiting.
(11) To be aware of the possibility of hyperglycaemia as a result of steroids, pain.
(12) Short-acting sulphonylureas or insulin may be indicated. Biguanides may be contraindicated if renal or hepatic failure is present.
(13) To monitor biochemistry results and report abnormal results.

Since the introduction of serotonin inhibitors (e.g. Ondansetron) to control nausea and vomiting these effects of anti-cancer therapy have decreased. Consequently there is less disruption of normal eating patterns.

Significant loss of vision

14.17 Key points

- Encourage independence.
- Maintain a safe environment.
- Orient patient to the environment and staff.
- Explain procedures fully.
- Return belongings to the same place.

People with diabetes have an increased risk of developing eye complications, leading to degrees of visual loss. Almost all Type 1 diabetics will eventually have eye complications to some degree.

14.18 Eye problems associated with diabetes

(1) The shape of the lens changes with blood glucose concentrations, leading to refractive changes and blurred vision. This usually corrects as the blood glucose is normalized, but may take some time.

(2) One-third of diabetics have retinopathy as a result of microvascular disease.

(3) People can have severe eye damage without being aware of it. Vision is not always affected. There is usually no pain or discomfort.

(4) Cataracts are more common in people with diabetes.

(5) Maculopathy is the most common cause of visual loss in diabetics.

(6) Sudden loss of vision is normally an emergency. It may be due to:
- vitreous haemorrhage
- retinal detachment
- retinal artery occlusion.

Reassurance, avoidance of stress and sudden movement, and urgent ophthalmological assessment are required.

(7) Prevention and early detection are important aspects in the management of this distressing complication, involving:
- good control of the diabetes
- regular eye examinations (commencing at diagnosis in Type 2 and within 5 years in Type 1)
- retinal photography
- fluorescein angiography.

14.19   Resources for people with visual impairment

People with significant visual loss often require assistance to perform blood glucose monitoring and to administer their own insulin. It is important to encourage independence as far as possible. Careful assessment is important and should include assessment of the home situation.

The Royal Society for the Blind offers a variety of services for people who have degrees of visual loss. These services include:

● Assessment of the home situation to determine if modifications are necessary to ensure safety at home.
● Low vision clinics.
● Talking library and books in braille.
● Training on how to cope in the community with deteriorating vision.

The Australian Commonwealth Government has made provision for people with corrected vision of less than 6/60 or tunnel vision, to receive a pension. The pension for the visually impaired entitles people to significant concessions, including transport. The Domiciliary and Visiting Nursing Services play a major role in maintaining visually impaired people in their own homes.

14.20   Aids for people with low vision

Various magnifying devices are available to help people continue to care for themselves. They can be obtained from diabetes associations and some pharmacies specializing in diabetic products. Other aids include:

(1) Insulin administration:
    ● clicking syringes, Instaject devices, insulin pens
    ● chest magnifying glass (available from some opticians); Magniguide – fits both 50 and 100 unit syringes and enlarges the markings
    ● location tray for drawing up insulin.
(2) Blood glucose monitoring:
    ● strip guides for accurate placement of the blood onto the strips
    ● talking blood glucose meters
    ● meters with large result display areas.

People with visual problems and/or red/green colour blindness may have difficulty interpreting the colours on visual test strips.

---

(3) Medications:
    ● dosette boxes which can be prefilled with the correct medication.

14.21 Nursing care of visually impaired patients

14.21.1 Aims of Care

- To encourage independence as far as possible.
- To ensure the environment is safe when the patient is mobile.

14.21.2 Patients confined to bed

(1) Introduce yourself and address the patient by name, so the patient is aware that you are talking to him/her.

(2) Ascertain how much the patient is able to see. (Few patients are totally blind.)

(3) Some patients prefer a corner bed because it makes location easier, avoids confusion with equipment belonging to other patients and enables greater ease in setting up personal belongings.

(4) Introduce the patient to their room mates.

(5) If you move the patient's belongings they must be returned to the same place.

(6) Explain all procedures carefully and fully before commencing. (An injection when you can't see it and don't expect it can be very unnerving.)

(7) If eye bandages are required make sure the ears and other sensory organs are not covered as well.

(8) Consider extra adjustable lighting for those patients with useful residual vision.

(9) Mark the patient's medication with large print labels or use a dosette.

(10) A radio, talking clock, talking watch, braille watch, or a large figured watch, helps the patient keep orientated to time and place.

(11) Indicate when you are leaving the room and concluding a conversation.

14.21.3 Patients who are mobile

(1) A central point (like the patient's bed) assists with orientating a patient to a room.

(2) When orientating a patient to a new area, walk with them until they become familiar with the route.

(3) Keep obstacles (trolleys, etc.) clear of pathways where possible.

14.21.4 Meal times

(1) Describe the menu and let the patient make a choice.

(2) Ensure the patient knows their meal has been delivered.

(3) Ask 'Do you need assistance with your meal?' rather than say, 'I will cut your meat for you.'
(4) Colour contrast is important for some patients. A white plate on a red tray-cloth may assist with location of place setting.

These guidelines have been adapted from *Guidelines for Health Professionals*, PRO 17, developed by the Royal Society For The Blind, Australia, and are reproduced with permission.

14.22   Further reading

Hills, S.H. (1986) Nutritional aspects of intensive care. In *Handbook of Critical Care Nursing*, (ed. K. Emanuelsen), Chapter 11. Wiley, New York.
Jung, R.T. & Sikora, K. (1984) *Endocrine Problems in Cancer*. Heinemann Medical Books, London.
Rovinski, C.A. & Zastocki, D.K. (1989) *Home Care*, Unit 11. W.B. Saunders, Philadelphia.

Chapter 15
Foot Care while in Hospital

15.1 Key points

- Assess feet thoroughly.
- Improve blood glucose control.
- Maintain safe environment.
- Report all abnormalities.
- Ensure foot care education.
- Refer to appropriate allied health professionals (diabetes educator, podiatrist).

Foot care is an extremely important aspect of the nursing care of people with diabetes in hospital. The combination of mechanical factors and vascular and nerve damage as a complication of diabetes leads to an increased risk of ulceration, infection and amputation.

It is estimated that 40% of diabetics have neuropathy and 20% of hospital admissions are for foot-related problems.

15.2 Vascular changes

(1) *Macrovascular* (major vessel disease) may lead to:
- intermittent claudication
- poor circulation to the lower limbs which leads to decreased nutrition, tissue hypoxia and delayed healing if any trauma occurs in this area; the injured tissue is prone to infection and gangrene may result.

(2) *Microvascular* (small vessel disease) leads to thickening of capillary basement membranes, poor blood supply to the skin and tissue hypoxia, predisposing the feet to infection and slow healing.

15.3 Neuropathy

Diabetic neuropathy is defined as the presence of clinical or subclinical evidence of peripheral nerve damage which cannot be attributed to any other disease process. Neuropathy may affect the sensory nerves resulting in pain, tingling, pins and needles or numbness. These symptoms are often worse at night. The sensory loss results in insensitivity to pain, cold, heat, touch and vibration. Trauma, pressure areas, sores, blisters, cuts and burns may not be detected by the patient. Callous formation, ulceration and bone involvement can occur.

The motor nerves may be affected, resulting in weakness, loss of muscle fibres and diminished reflexes. Both types of nerves can be affected at the same time. Medications are not very effective in the treatment of neuropathy, but some commonly used drugs include analgesics, such as nonsteroidal anti-inflammatory drugs, anti-depressants, anti-convulsants and capsaician cream. Experimental drugs include the aldose reductase inhibitors such as Tolrestat.

The autonomic nervous system may also be affected by diabetes. Autonomic nervous system involvement may lead to an absence of sweating, which causes dry, cracked skin and increases the risk of infection. Other effects of autonomic neuropathy include gastric stasis, impotence, hypoglycaemic unawareness and incontinence.

The small muscle wasting secondary to longstanding neuropathy may lead to abnormal foot shapes, e.g. clawing of the toes, making the purchase of well fitting shoes difficult.

Vascular disease, neuropathy and infection are more likely to develop if there is longstanding hyperglycaemia (poor diabetic control), which con-

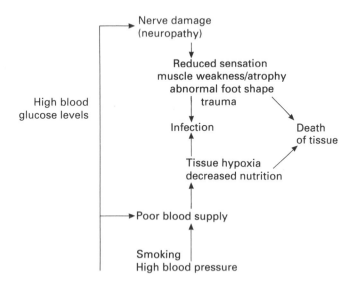

Fig. 15.1 Diagrammatic representation of the factors leading to foot problems in people with diabetes.

tributes to the accumulation of sorbitol through the polyol pathway, leading to damage to the nerves and small blood vessels. Figure 15.1 illustrates the interaction of factors leading to foot problems in people with diabetes.

Table 15.1 lists changes in feet due to the normal aging process, and Table 15.2 lists the risk factors for the development of foot problems in people with diabetes. These factors should all be incorporated in the nursing assessment to ensure that appropriate foot care is part of the overall management of the patient.

Table 15.1   Changes in feet due to normal aging.

(1) Skin becomes thin, fragile
(2) Nails thick and often deformed
(3) Blood supply is reduced
(4) Nerve function often impaired
(5) Muscle weakness and wasting
(6) Arthritis, may lead to pain and deformity

Table 15.2   Risk factors for the development of foot problems in people with diabetes.

(1) Diabetes, especially if blood glucose is continually high
(2) Smoking
(3) Obesity
(4) High blood pressure
(5) Cardiac disease
(6) Lack of or inadequate foot care
(7) Inappropriate footwear
(8) Delay in seeking help
(9) Previous foot problems

15.4   Objectives of care

(1) To identify feet most at risk of trauma, ulceration and infection during hospitalization by assessing vascular, nerve and diabetic status.
(2) To assess patient knowledge of foot care.
(3) To reinforce appropriate preventative foot care.
(4) To prevent trauma, infection and pressure areas developing while in hospital.
(5) To treat any problem detected.

(6) To refer to podiatry, orthotics, physiotherapy, rehabilitation, diabetes educator as necessary.
(7) To control or eliminate any factors which predisposes the patient to the risk of foot problems in hospital.

15.5 Nursing responsibilities

(1) To assess the feet carefully on admission. Assess self-care potential (can the patient reach the feet, see clearly?). When assessing the feet, obtain information about:
(a) Past medical history:
- glycaemic control
- previous foot-related problems/deformities
- smoking habits
- nerve and vascular related risk factors
- claudication, rest pain
- alcohol intake.
(b) Type of footwear (socks, shoes):
- hygiene
- activity level.
(c) Social factors:
- living alone
- elderly.
(2) When examining the feet:
- check pulses, dorsalis pedis, posterior tibial
- assess toenails: thick, layered, curved, ingrowing toenails will need attention
- note foot structure; overlapping toes.
(3) Note also:
- pallor on elevation of leg
- capillary return (normally 1–2 seconds)
- any discoloration of legs
- hair loss.
(4) To ensure appropriate foot hygiene:
- wash in lukewarm water
- check water temperature with wrist before putting the patient into a bath
- dry thoroughly, including between toes
- apply cream to prevent dryness and cracks (urea cream, sorbelene).
(5) Ensure Elastoplast/Band Aids, bandages do *not* encircle toes as they can act like tourniquets and cut off circulation.

    (6) Maintain a safe environment:
- use a bead cradle
- ensure shoes are worn if walking around the ward
- strict bed rest may be necessary while the ulcer is healing
- maintain aseptic technique.

    (7) Check feet daily and report any changes or the development of any callus, abrasion or trauma.

    (8) Monitor blood glucose control.

    (9) Attend to dressings and administer antibiotics according to treatment order. Antibiotics are often given intravenously.

  (10) Ensure preventative foot care education is provided, to give the patient with diabetes:
- an understanding of effects of diabetes on the feet
- a knowledge of appropriate footwear
- the ability to identify foot risk factors
- an understanding of the principle effects of poor control (continual hyperglycaemia) on foot health
- knowledge about the services available for assistance with their diabetes care and how to obtain advice about foot care
- knowledge about appropriate foot care practices, in particular that they must inspect their feet daily and seek help early if any problems are found.

15.6   Classification of foot ulcers

Foot ulcers can be loosely classified as:

(1) Clean, superficial ulcer.
(2) Deeper ulcer, possibly infected, but no bone involvement.
(3) Deep ulcer, tracking infection and bone involvement.
(4) Localized gangrene and necrosis (usually forefoot, heel).
(5) Extensive gangrene of foot.

    The depth and width of the ulcer should be recorded regularly; a plastic template dated and filed in the patient's history aids in the assessment of changes in ulcer size. The presence, amount and type of exudate must be recorded.

    Painting the area with a betadine or other skin antiseptic is of little value. Coloured antiseptics can obscure some of the signs of infection.

    Dressings may be needed to absorb the exudate and protect the foot. Surgical debridement, amputation or an occlusive dressing may be required. It is important to keep the dressing moist and the pH acidic to promote healing. The moisture aids in pain relief, decreases the healing time and gives a better cosmetic result. An acidic environment promotes

Table 15.3 Management of specific foot problems while in hospital.

Problem	Treatment
Burning, paraesthesia, aching	Encourage person to walk Maintain euglycaemia
Pain	Foot cradle, sheepskin, medications as ordered
Dry skin, cracks	Clean, dry carefully, apply moisturizer, e.g. urea cream, sorbelene
Claudication	Medications as ordered Rest Elevate feet Vascular assessment Angiography
Foot deformity	Consult podiatrist Physiotherapy Orthotist
Ulcers, infection	Refer to specific medical order Assess daily Make template to note change in size of ulcer Antibiotics See classification of foot ulcers, section 15.6 Debridement, amputation

granulation tissue. The management in hospital of ulcers and other specific foot problems is listed in Table 15.3.

Note: healing of diabetic foot ulcers is slow and bed rest is important. The patient may be otherwise well. Encourage independence with blood glucose testing and insulin administration. Refer for occupational therapy.

Careful discharge planning is imperative:

● To ensure mobilization and rehabilitation.
● Interim placement in an extended care facility may be necessary.
● Assess the physical and social support available after discharge.

Orthopaedic patients with foot or leg plasters should be encouraged *not* to scratch under the plaster, especially if they have 'at risk' feet. Damage can occur and remain undetected until the plaster is removed.

15.7   Further reading

Kozak, G., Hoar, C., Rowbotham, J. *et al.* (1984) *Management of Diabetic Foot Problems*. W.B. Saunders, Philadelphia.
Pamphlets from pharmaceutical companies and some diabetic units on care of the diabetic foot.

Chapter 16
Diabetes in Children, Pregnancy and the Elderly

Diabetes in children, during pregnancy and in the elderly can present special problems which should be considered when formulating nursing care plans. This chapter briefly outlines particular areas where extra care and nursing vigilance is important for these groups of people.

16.1 Diabetes in children and adolescents

Diabetes occurring in children and adolescents is usually Type 1, with a sudden onset of symptoms and requiring insulin injections for survival. Insulin and dietary requirements can change rapidly, especially in children, due to rapid changes in activity levels. Therefore consistent acceptable blood glucose levels may be difficult to achieve.

A supportive and encouraging family is important if the child is to accept diabetes and eventually take over diabetic self-management. The family in turn needs support, advice and encouragement.

During adolescence the hormonal surge at puberty can make blood glucose control difficult. Dietary restrictions and the diabetic regime can be seen as obstacles to fitting in with peer activities and may be neglected. Achieving independence from the family can be difficult.

The transfer from paediatric care to adult specialist care can be very stressful. Neglect of the diabetes, failure to attend appointments and poor control are not uncommon. Tact and understanding are very important if these young people are not to be lost to adequate medical supervision.

16.1.1 Management goals

(1) To achieve normal growth and development.
(2) To prevent or delay the onset of diabetes-related complications.
(3) To ensure a balanced diet.
(4) To promote acceptance of the diabetes by the child and the family.
(5) To assist the child to gradually take over the self-care tasks.
(6) To transfer to adult care.

16.1.2   Nursing responsibilities

In addition to those nursing tasks outlined in specific chapters it is important to:

- Document height and weight on percentile charts.
- Encourage independence and allow the child to inject and test if already
  doing so.
- Monitor dietary intake and ensure appropriate dietary review by
  dietitian.
- Ensure diabetic knowledge is assessed.
- Ensure privacy during procedures.
- Avoid admitting adolescents and children to wards with elderly people, if
  possible.

16.2   Diabetes and pregnancy

Diabetes may occur during pregnancy (gestational diabetes; see section
1.3.3). Most women are screened for diabetes during pregnancy so that
blood glucose levels can be controlled to avoid the risks having diabetes
places on both mother and baby. Women particularly at risk are those with
a history of diabetes in the family, diabetes during a previous pregnancy or
previous delivery of a large baby.

Blood glucose levels may return to normal after delivery, however the
possibility of diabetes manifesting again in later life is increased, as are the
risks of developing long-term diabetic complications. Pre-pregnancy
counselling and achieving good control is important for the women with
existing diabetes, contemplating pregnancy.

Regular appointments with the obstetrician and diabetologist and close
fetal monitoring are very important. Care of the mother and baby during
labour and delivery are specialty areas and outside the scope of this
manual.

16.2.1   Management goals

(1) To achieve good blood glucose control before becoming pregnant to
    decrease the possibility of:
    - stillbirth
    - prematurity
    - fetal abnormalities
    - macrosomia
    - respiratory distress
    - Caesarian section.

(2) To maintain good blood glucose control during pregnancy (4–5 mmol/l, i.e. normal).
(3) To provide adequate carbohydrate intake to avoid ketonaemia, especially during the second trimester.
(4) To provide adequate nutrient intake to allow normal growth and development of the baby without compromising the mother's health.
(5) To monitor kidney function and screen for pre-eclampsia and hydramnios.
(6) To monitor maternal weight.
(8) To encourage no smoking and limited alcohol consumption.
(9) To deliver the baby before 38 weeks usually.

OHAs should not be used during pregnancy. People with Type 2 diabetes often require insulin during pregnancy.

Important points concerning pregnancy in a patient with existing diabetes:

- The risk of the child developing diabetes is relatively low.
- Babies of diabetic mothers who maintain normal blood glucose levels throughout pregnancy are less likely to develop congenital abnormalities.
- If the patient is taking OHAs prior to pregnancy, the doctor will change the treatment to insulin during pregnancy.
- OHAs prior to pregnancy do not prevent the mother breast feeding her baby as long as she remains on insulin.

16.3 Diabetes in the elderly

Elderly people with diabetes often have multiple health problems, some of which are the result of diabetes-related complications. There may also be a self-care deficit and decreased mental functioning. Elderly people require specific nursing care to decrease the risk of additional problems occurring as a result of hospitalization.

Age, life expectancy, other health problems and the social situation should be taken into consideration when planning the care of elderly diabetic patients. Obtaining near normal blood glucose tests and preventing the long-term complications of diabetes may not be priority treatment aims. It is important to control uncomfortable symptoms (polyuria, polydipsia, lethargy) and to ensure that the risk of hypoglycaemia is minimal. The particular problems which may be encountered in elderly diabetics are detailed in Table 16.1.

Table 16.1 Special problems of the elderly diabetic.

Problem	Risk
Hyperglycaemia	Hyperosmolar coma Ketoacidosis Thrombosis
Poor food intake	Hypoglycaemia Trauma
Cerebral insufficiency	Stroke Non-recognition of hypos Trauma
Cardiac insufficiency	Myocardial infarction Confusion
Autonomic neuropathy	Urinary tract infections Unrecognized hypoglycaemia Myocardial infarction
Peripheral insufficiency	Foot ulcers, claudication
Peripheral neuropathy	Unstable gait, ulcers
Visual loss	Self-care problems/insulin administration, BG testing
Skin atrophy	Pressure sores Trauma
Communication problems, e.g. hearing loss	Misunderstandings Stress
Stress	High blood pressure levels High blood glucose

In addition, degrees of dementia may make assessment of hypo/hyperglycaemia difficult. Polypharmacy can be responsible for undesirable drug interactions. Hypoglycaemia occurring in elderly people managed with OHAs can be difficult to recognize clinically. The usual signs and symptoms may not be present (see Chapter 8). Presentation may resemble a cerebrovascular accident or mental confusion. Hypoglycaemia may be more profound and prolonged or become chronic. Check blood glucose of elderly people presenting with these possible diagnoses, especially in the emergency department.

16.4   Further reading

Ashwell, S. (1992) *Diabetes and Aging: A Guide to Management Education*. Graphic Type, Sydney.
Court, J. (1991) *Modern Living with Diabetes*. Diabetes Australia, Victoria.

Chapter 17
Outline of the Psychological Issues Related to Having Diabetes

---

17.1 Key points

- Initial denial of diabetes is common.
- Assess factors which influence acceptance of diabetes.
- Repeated admissions for DKA or hypoglycaemia may indicate an underlying psychosocial problem.
- Avoid labels such as 'non-compliant' or 'a diabetic'.
- Offer support, respect and encouragement.

This chapter is a brief outline only, of the psychological aspects of having diabetes. Reactions to the diagnosis of diabetes are unique to the individual concerned, however several common reactions have been documented. They include: anger, guilt, fear, helplessness, confusion, relief and denial. A knowledge of some of the issues involved will enable nursing staff to understand the difficulties associated with living with diabetes.

Many factors will influence how a person accepts the diagnosis of diabetes and assumes responsibility for self-care. These factors include:

- Age.
- Existing knowledge about diabetes.
- Health beliefs.
- Locus of control.

A period of grief and denial is normal. Figure 17.1 is one model of the 'diabetic grief cycle' loosely based on Helen Kubler Ross's work, associated with death and dying. Lack of knowledge, or inaccurate knowledge about diabetes, produces stress and anxiety. The invisible nature of the condition (in Type 2 diabetes there are often no presenting symptoms), can lead to disbelief and denial of the diagnosis. Denial is appropriate early in the course of the disease and enables people to maintain a positive attitude and cope with the altered health status.

Adequate time must be allowed for the person to grieve for the losses he/she perceives to be associated with diabetes (loss of spontaneity, life-style) and a changed body image. However, prolonged denial can inhibit

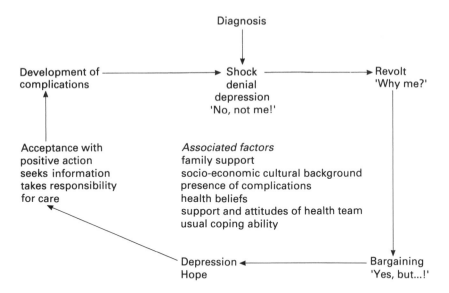

Acceptance of diabetes varies from months to years.
Some people never accept diabetes.
The development of complications means another readjustment.

Fig. 17.1 Model of the diabetic grief cycle.

appropriate self-care; cause people to ignore warning signs of other problems; and may lead to failure to attend medical appointments.

Acceptance of diabetes involves dealing with:

- Pain.
- Hospitalization, medical staff.
- Lifelong treatment.
- Body image changes.
- Friends/family relationships.
- Fluctuating blood glucose levels.
- Emotional lability.
- Loss of independence.

The tasks required to maintain acceptable blood glucose control are tedious and sometimes painful. There are financial costs involved which can be a burden for some people (insulin, testing equipment, doctors' visits, increased insurance premiums). They add to the stress associated with having a disease no-one wanted in the first place.

There is no holiday from diabetes for the patient.

Diabetes has a 'bad reputation' in the community, with many associated myths (e.g. 'eating sugar causes diabetes') which must be discussed and dispelled. Such myths can be associated with self-blame and guilt feelings. In addition, social pressures make denial of the diabetes and failure to follow medical advice easy. 'A little piece of cake won't hurt you.'

17.2   Type 1 diabetes

Diabetes diagnosed in childhood can produce enormous guilt and anxiety for the child and the parents. Marital strife is not uncommon and is often exacerbated by the diabetes. The parents must learn how to care for the child at the same time as coping with their own feelings. Inflicting pain on a child (injections, blood tests) is very difficult to do, and such tasks often fall to the mother.

Eventually the parents must allow the child to care for his/her own diabetes. It can be extremely difficult for the parents to 'let go' and therefore for the child to achieve independence. Other children in the family may feel deprived of attention. Sweets, the traditional reward for good behaviour, are often withdrawn and this may be seen as a punishment.

Some childhood behaviour such as irritability and awkwardness can be difficult to distinguish from hypoglycaemia, making management difficult. Hypoglycaemia itself is feared and hated by children and parents and mostly underrated by health care staff. It is not unknown for people to run blood glucose levels high to avoid hypoglycaemia.

As the child matures and develops they need to take over the care of their diabetes. It can be difficult for the parent to 'let go'. There may be concerns about passing diabetes to their own children in the future. Support, encouragement and referral for counselling if necessary are vital aspects of diabetes care.

Diabetes is the perfect disease for manipulating others and gaining attention. Withholding insulin can result in ketoacidosis, with the mobilization of family, friends and health resources. Hypoglycaemia can have the same effect. Repeated admissions for hypoglycaemia or DKA need to be investigated carefully and diplomatically.

17.3   Type 2 diabetes

The diagnosis of diabetes in later life means the person may need to change behaviours developed over years. Eating patterns often have to be modified. Restrictions are often resented with resultant anger, denial or neglect. Alternatively the patient may meticulously follow the management plan.

Knowledge about possible diabetic complications or the development of complications leads to stress, which in turn contributes to elevated blood glucose levels. Relationships may be disrupted as in Type 1 diabetes, with families/spouses becoming over-protective, resulting in over-dependence or rebelliousness.

People tend to cope better and manage the self-care tasks more easily if the family is supportive, yet allows independence.

17.4 Compliance/non-compliance

These terms are judgemental, prejudiced and negative in nature. They are labels best avoided in relation to diabetic self-care tasks. Failure to comply with one aspect of care does not necessarily indicate complete neglect of the diabetes. In fact, forgetting and omitting aspects of care is probably 'normal' behaviour and obsessive attention to routine may indicate fear and anxiety.

It is important to establish why the particular task is neglected. Reasons include:

- Unreal expectations of the staff resulting from a lack of knowledge of the person's capabilities and social situation.
- Setting of health professional rather than patient goals.
- Lack of knowledge of what is required.
- Lack of understanding as a result of poor communication.
- Inadequate support from family/friends and the health care team.
- Health beliefs and attitudes of the patient.
- Physical disabilities such as low vision, and diminished fine motor skills.
- Patient 'burn out'.
- Financial difficulties.

17.4.1 Patient requirements

- To be treated as normal.
- To be treated as a person, not 'a diabetic'.
- To be trusted and accepted.
- To know how and where to obtain advice.

Support, encouragement and focusing on positive achievements are far more helpful than 'shame and blame'.

Achievable goals should be negotiated with the patient. It is the patient's expectations which will be met rather than those of the health professional. It is important to recognize that diabetes is never easy. 'Good' and 'bad' when referring to blood glucose levels are judgemental terms. Substitute 'high' and 'low'. Some people resent being called 'a diabetic'. It is preferable to say 'a person with diabetes'.

Some patients express concern about being admitted to hospital, over and above the usual reactions to illness/hospitalization. They feel abnormal by being singled out for special meals and having labels such as 'diabetic diet' attached to the bed. They are sometimes made to feel incompetent when they have often been caring for their diabetes for years. For example, when requesting sugar to avoid hypoglycaemia, not being allowed to test blood glucose or to give own injections.

Some people feel that they are blamed if they are admitted with a diabetic complication. They 'should have known better' and taken care of their diabetes better. Patients become frustrated when they are labelled 'non-compliant'. Continuous negative feedback only reinforces that the person is not coping. Learned helplessness can result.

17.5   Further reading

Dunning, P. (1991) Why counsel the patient and family with Type 2 diabetes? *Treating Diabetes*, 5.

Horn, B. (1990) *Living with Diabetes*. Houghton, Victoria.

Lubkin, I.M. (1990) *Chronic Illness Impact and Interventions*. Jones and Bartlett, Boston.

Raymond, M. (1992) *The Human Side of Diabetes: Beyond Doctors, Diet, Drugs*. Noble Press, Chicago.

Chapter 18
Diabetes Education

18.1 Key points

- Written instructions should be provided.
- Information should be supplied in 'chunks'.
- Information must be culturally relevant.
- Information should be supplied according to individual needs.
- Regular knowledge assessment is important.
- Information must be consistent with that taught by the diabetes team.

18.2 Introduction

Diabetes education is an integral part of the management of diabetes. The overall goal of diabetes education is to assist the patient to accept and integrate the diabetes management tasks successfully into their lifestyle and self-concept, in order to achieve and maintain optimum diabetic control.

There are standardized patient education guidelines, but each patient should be assessed and a teaching plan developed to ensure individual learning needs are addressed. Diabetes education is often divided into:

- Survival skills: that information necessary to be safe at home.
- Basic knowledge: that information which will enable greater understanding about diabetes and its care.
- Ongoing education: the continued acquisition of new knowledge, including changes in technology and management practices applicable to self-care.

18.2.1 Survival skills

Survival skills are taught at diagnosis and should be reviewed regularly. The family should be involved whenever possible. Minimal information for safety is given and written information supplied. However, specific concerns/questions of the patient should be addressed. The patient should be able to:

- Demonstrate correct insulin care and administration techniques.
- Know the effect of medications and food on blood glucose levels.
- Know the names of their insulin/tablets.
- Demonstrate correct monitoring techniques (blood and/or urine testing) and appropriate documentation of the results.
- Know the significance of ketones in the urine (Type 1).
- Recognize the signs and symptoms, causes and appropriate treatment of hypoglycaemia.
- Know that regular meals containing the appropriate amount of carbohydrate are important.
- Have an emergency contact telephone number if help is required.
- Demonstrate safe disposal of sharps.

The diabetic education record in Patient Care Sheet 4 is an example of the type of form used to document 'survival information' and plan for further teaching.

18.2.2 Ongoing education

Education can be continued on an individual basis or in group programmes. As education is a lifelong process both systems are usually employed. Survival information should be reviewed and further information given. The patient should gradually be able to:

- Demonstrate appropriate insulin adjustment considering the effects of food, activity and medication on blood glucose.
- Know the appropriate management of illnesses at home, especially to continue insulin/diabetes tablets, to continue to drink fluids and to test the urine for ketones, especially Type 1.
- Recognize the signs and symptoms of hypoglycaemia and treat appropriately.
- Cope in special situations, such as eating out, during travel and playing sports, in terms of medication and food intake.
- Know that appropriate foot care will help prevent foot problems and hospital admissions.
- Know that good diabetic control and regular examination of the eyes, feet, blood pressure, cardiovascular system and kidney function can prevent or delay the development of long-term diabetic complications.
- Know that certain jobs and activities are unsuitable for people with diabetes on insulin, e.g. scuba diving, driving heavy vehicles.
- Accept the wisdom of wearing some form of medical alert system identifying them as having diabetes.

PATIENT CARE SHEET 4:
DIABETIC EDUCATION RECORD CHART

DIABETIC EDUCATION RECORD

Date of referral ....

Referred by Dr/Rn ....

Unit ....

Ward/Op ....

Language spoken at home ....

Understanding of English: good/fair/poor ....

Other communication problems ....

Method used to address problem ....

Indicate perceived level of skill and understanding attained ....

Follow-up requirements ....

Information Supplied

(1)   What is diabetes? ....

(2)   How it is controlled:

    •   diet ....

    •   tablets/insulin ....

(3)   Urine testing - renal threshold ....

(4)   Home glucose monitoring ....

(5)   Diet and nutrition ....

(6)   Insulin and tablets:

    •   care of ....

    •   drawing up and giving injection ....

    •   when to take tablets/insulin ....

    •   sharps disposal ....

(7)   Hypos ....   (8)   Sick days ....

(9)   Foot care ....   (10) Sport & exercise ....

(11) Dentist ....   (12) Travel & driving ....

PATIENT CARE SHEET 4 *contd*

Other information discussed ....

Family support: good/fair/poor ....

Domiciliary Instructions ....

....

....

Patient Discharge Checklist

(1)   Education material - itemise ....

(2)   Record book ....

(3)   Blood testing equipment - type ....

(4)   Urine testing ....   (5)   Diet chart ....

(6)   Diabetic card complete ....

(7)   Starter pack syringes/needles/monolets ....

(8)   Discharged to: diabetic clinic/LMO/specialist ....

(9)   Referred for further education ....

Enrolment in Diabetic Association ....

Signature of Registered Nurse ....   Date ....

Consistency of information given by various members of the health care team is important to avoid confusion.

18.3   Special issues

Questions should be addressed as they arise and planned into teaching programmes as appropriate to the individual. Questions may relate to:

- Pregnancy and diabetes.
- Sexuality and diabetes.
- Exercise.
- Weight control.

It is not absolutely necessary for people with diabetes to have a detailed knowledge about the causes and pathophysiology of diabetes in order to achieve good control.

18.4   The role of the bedside nurse in diabetes education

Patient teaching is an independent nursing function and education is a vital part of the diabetic treatment plan. Therefore the teaching of patients by the bedside nurse is well within the scope of professional nursing practice. Some key points should be kept in mind when talking to people with diabetes:

(1) Consider the psychological and social aspects when discussing diabetes.
(2) Encourage questions and dialogue.
(3) Ask open questions.
(4) Teach specific skills and allow the patient time to practise new skills (e.g. insulin administration).
(5) Allow time for patients to discuss difficulties and concerns about diabetes.
(6) Relate new information to the patient's experience.

Bedside teaching can allow for teaching at a 'teachable moment' and effective reinforcement of information. It must be consistent with diabetes team teaching and hospital policies/procedures. The nurse must have the appropriate knowledge.

Diabetes education makes a substantial contribution to the health and well-being of the patient, allowing them to participate in decision making about their care in hospital, and to make appropriate decisions at home.

Teaching in the ward effectively reinforces the information supplied by the diabetes educator, doctor, podiatrist and dietitian. However, ward teaching *must* be consistent with that of the diabetes team and procedures such as insulin technique and blood glucose monitoring performed correctly according to the diabetic protocols. Patients are quick to perceive inconsistencies and may become confused, or have their faith in the staff undermined. Some examples of relevant Patient Instruction Sheets will be found at the end of this chapter.

Learning is facilitated when the need/readiness to learn is perceived and immediately applied in a given situation: that is, 'teaching at a teachable moment'. Teachable moments often occur when the ward staff are performing routine nursing care, such as blood glucose tests, or giving injections.

Teaching is non-verbal as well as verbal. People learn by observation, therefore the nurse is a role model and care should be taken to perform procedures correctly and to refer questions to another person if the answer is not known. In this way, formal and informal ongoing education in the ward is possible and desirable. The nurse's own knowledge about diabetes will influence his/her willingness and ability to participate in patient teaching. Theories of teaching and learning were not traditionally part of the nurse training. This is changing with the advent of college-based training and the focus on preventative health care.

Many factors can influence teaching and learning. Some of these are shown in Table 18.1. It is the responsibility of the teacher to ensure that the environment is not distracting. Noise in a busy ward can make conversation difficult and hinder learning. The patient should be as comfortable as possible and free from pain.

Table 18.1   **Factors which influence teaching and learning.**

Factor	Patient	Nurse
Health beliefs	✓	✓
Social support	✓	
Well-being/illness	✓	
Environment	✓	✓
Knowledge	✓	✓
Skills	✓	✓
Time	✓	✓
Perceived responsibility		✓
Work priority		✓
Perception of teaching role		✓

The following basic principles need to be considered when planning a teaching session:

- The aim of the session.
- The patient's needs/goals.
- Objectives should be realistic and achievable.
- The environment must be conducive to learning.
- Ascertain and build on the patient's knowledge.
- Relate teaching to patient's experience.
- Demonstrate skills to be acquired.
- Provide opportunity for the patient to practise skill.
- Evaluate the skill and knowledge.
- Provide positive reinforcement.
- Review information before commencing next teaching session.

It is usual to begin with the simple concepts and proceed to more complex ones.

Patient Instruction Sheets 3 to 7 are examples of patient information material used in teaching. They are often available in several languages. In some cases the medical terms may need to be replaced with the patient's words. Blood glucose monitoring is discussed in Chapter 4. Specific patient instruction will depend on the testing system being used.

18.5   Insulin administration

Insulin may be administered using an insulin syringe, an insulin pen or an insulin pump.

18.5.1   Insulin syringes

Insulin syringes come in three sizes:

(1) 50 units (see Fig. 18.1): each line marking on the 50 unit syringe is equal to 1 unit of insulin. Fifty unit syringes are used for small doses of insulin (<50 units).
(2) 100 units (see Fig. 18.2): each line marking on the 100 unit syringe is equal to 2 units of insulin. One hundred unit syringes are used for large doses of insulin (>50 units).
(3) 30 units (see Fig. 18.3): a 30 unit syringe is available for paediatric use.

18.5.2   Insulin pump (continuous subcutaneous insulin infusion)

Insulin is constantly infused through a fine needle and tubing inserted under the skin and left in place. A bolus of insulin is given before each meal. There are several brands of pump available with different features, and

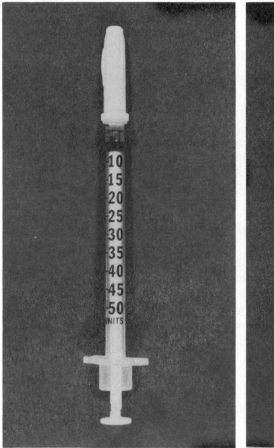

Fig. 18.1 50 unit syringe.

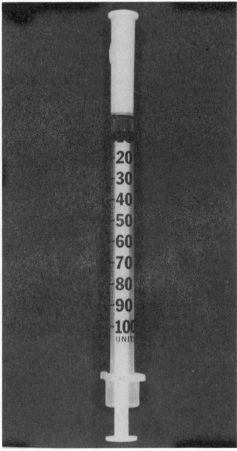

Fig. 18.2 100 unit syringe.

they are expensive. The patient must understand the use and care of the pump and be prepared to test the blood glucose at least four times each day. Figure 18.4 illustrates a typical infusion pump.

18.5.3 Insulin pens

There are several insulin pens (see Fig. 18.5) available. They consist of:

- A detachable needle (the same size as on the insulin syringe).
- A section to hold the insulin penfill and a lid to protect the needle when not in use.

With some pens the total dose of insulin can be dialled and given by

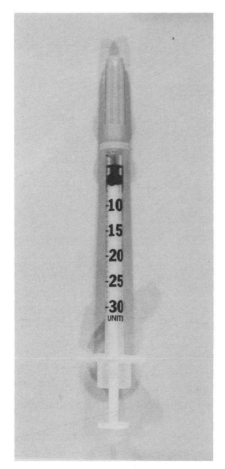

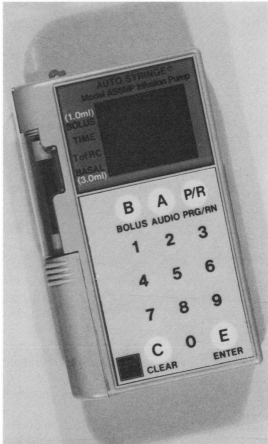

Fig. 18.3 30 unit syringe.   **Fig. 18.4** Insulin pump.

pushing a button. A second type of pen administers 2 units of insulin each time the button is depressed. Pens offer the advantage of being discreet and are often used by patients on basal bolus regimes, those who travel frequently and those who have difficulty drawing insulin into a syringe.

18.6   Guidelines for instructing patients about insulin pens

18.6.1   Patient Learning Requirements

The patient should be familiar with the structure and function of the particular insulin pen chosen. They must be able to:

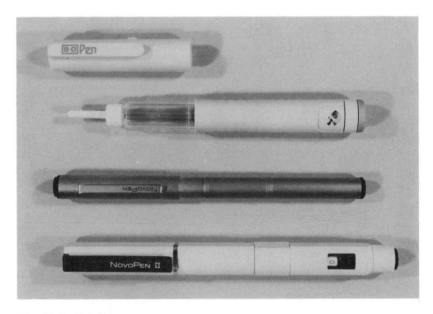

Fig. 18.5   Insulin pens.

- Assemble the pen in the correct sequence.
- Load the insulin penfill correctly.
- Ensure insulin is expelled from the needle after loading the penfill.
- Know how many units are contained in the penfill and when to replace the penfill.
- Know how to inject the insulin according to the particular pen chosen (for example, one depression of the plunger of Novo Pen 1 delivers 2 units of insulin).
- Know how to store and transport the pen.
- Know the appropriate method of cleaning and maintaining the pen.
- Recognize signs that the device may be malfunctioning and know what action to take to remedy the situation.

Note: it is recommended that a supply of insulin syringes and one bottle of insulin be kept for emergencies.

18.6.2   Suggested protocol for commencing pen use

(1) Begin the new regime during a stable metabolic period.
(2) Test HbA1c, cholesterol and triglycerides before commencing the new regime, and then 3 to 6 months later.
(3) Assess patient knowledge about:
   - hypoglycaemia

- sport
- sick day care
- travel
- eating out
- blood glucose monitoring.

(4) Educate or re-educate as necessary. Blood glucose monitoring should be performed four or five times each day until stabilized onto the new regime (2 to 3 weeks).

(5) Review progress in 1 week and keep contact by telephone until blood glucose is stable and in the appropriate range.

It is important to discuss, and advise about, safe disposal of used equipment with the patient, especially sharps disposal at home. The guidelines for sharps disposal in the home can be found in section 21.14.1.

Example Patient Instruction Sheets

These Instruction Sheets are designed to be used with a practical demonstration of the procedure/s. They should not be handed out without adequate discussion. **They are examples only**.

PATIENT INSTRUCTION SHEET 3:
HOW TO DRAW UP INSULIN – ONE BOTTLE ONLY

HOW TO DRAW UP INSULIN - ONE BOTTLE ONLY

Your insulin is called ....

(1)   Remove insulin bottle from fridge. Check expiry date - do not use if exceeded.

   Cloudy insulin must be mixed before drawing up.

(2)   Gently invert insulin bottle or roll between hands until well mixed **(do not shake)**. Insulin should be "milky"; there should be no lumps.

   Clear insulin should be clear and colourless.

(3)   Clean bottle top with spirit.

(4)   Draw back plunger to .... units of air.

(5)   Inject air into insulin bottle, invert bottle and draw back .... units of insulin, ensuring that all air bubbles are removed from the syringe.

(6)   Administer insulin.

PATIENT INSTRUCTION SHEET 4:
HOW TO DRAW UP INSULIN – TWO BOTTLES

HOW TO DRAW UP INSULIN - TWO BOTTLES

Your insulins are called .... (clear)

.... (cloudy)

(1)   Remove insulin bottles from fridge. Check expiry date - do not use if exceeded.

(2)   Gently invert or roll bottle of "cloudy" insulin between hands, until "milky" **(do not shake)**.

(3)   Clean bottle tops with spirit.

(4)   Draw back plunger to .... units of air.

(5)   Inject air into cloudy insulin and remove needle from the bottle.

(6)   Draw back plunger to .... units of air.

(7)   Inject air into clear insulin.

(8)   Invert bottle and draw back .... units of clear insulin, ensuring that all air bubbles are removed from syringe.

(9)   Put needle into cloudy bottle and withdraw .... units of cloudy insulin to the <u>exact</u> required dose of the syringe.

(10)   If more cloudy insulin is accidently drawn up, discard contents of the syringe and start again.

(11)   Total clear and cloudy insulin equals .... units.

PATIENT INSTRUCTION SHEET 5:
HOW TO GIVE AN INSULIN INJECTION

HOW TO GIVE AN INSULIN INJECTION

1.   Insulin can be injected into the abdomen, thighs, buttock or upper arm. The abdomen is the preferred site.

2.   Inject into a different site each time.

3.   Pinch up a fold of skin between two fingers.

4.   Quickly push the needle into the skin at right angles.

5.   Gently push the plunger all the way to inject your insulin.

6.   Pull the syringe out quickly and apply pressure to the injection site.

Insulin should be stored away from heat and light. The bottle in use can be kept at room temperature. Stores should be kept in the refrigerator.

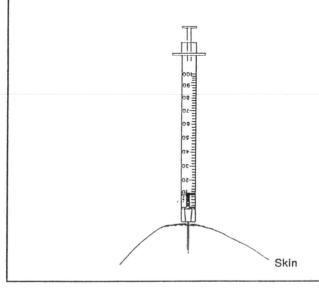

Skin

PATIENT INSTRUCTION SHEET 6:
HOW TO TEST URINE USING 'DIASTIX'

HOW TO TEST URINE USING "DIASTIX"

Diastix serve to examine the quantity of sugar in the urine.

Please test urine ....
(specify times)

Always ensure lid to bottle is screwed on tightly after removing test strip.

(1)　Wet blue pad on end of stick with urine by either:

　　　•　　dipping in stream of urine while voiding

　　　•　　collecting urine in container and dipping stick into this.

(2)　Tap edge of stick to remove excess urine.

(3)　Wait for 30 seconds.

(4)　Compare strip with colours on Diastix bottle.

(5)　Write results in your record book.

	0	trace	+	++	+++	++++
OR						
	0	trace	1/4%	1/2%	1%	2%

PATIENT INSTRUCTION SHEET 7(A): MANAGING YOUR DIABETES WHEN YOU ARE ILL: PATIENTS WITH TYPE 1 DIABETES

MANAGING YOUR DIABETES WHEN YOU ARE ILL

Illness (such as colds and flu) cause the body to make hormones which help the body fight the illness. These hormones usually also cause the blood glucose to go high. High blood glucose levels can lead to unpleasant symptoms like thirst, tiredness and passing a lot of urine.

By taking some simple precautions the minor illness can usually be treated at home.

What to Do

(1)   Continue to take your insulin. You may need to increase the dose during illness to control the blood glucose and prevent ketones from developing.

(2)   Test your blood glucose every 2-4 hours. Write down the test results.

(3)   Test your urine for ketones. If moderate to heavy ketones are detected consult your doctor.

(4)   Continue to drink fluids or eat if possible (see recommended food list).

(5)   Read the labels on any medication you take to treat the illness because it may contain sugar, sugar substitutes or other ingredients which cause the blood glucose to go high.

(6)   Rest.

(7)   Keep the phone number of your doctor or diabetes educator beside the telephone.

PATIENT INSTRUCTION SHEET 7(A) *contd*

When to Call the Doctor

(1)   If you have diarrhoea and/or vomiting.

(2)   If ketones develop in your urine.

(3)   If the blood glucose continues to rise.

(4)   If you develop signs of dehydration (loss of skin tone, sunken eyes, dry mouth).

(5)   If the illness does not get better in 2-3 days.

(6)   If you feel you need advice.

What to Tell the Doctor When You Call

(1)   How long you have been sick.

(2)   What the blood glucose level is.

(3)   How long the blood glucose has been high.

(4)   How many ketones are in the urine.

(5)   How frequently you are passing urine and how much.

(6)   If you are thirsty, tired or have a temperature.

(7)   What medications you have taken to treat the illness.

(8)   If you have vomiting or diarrhoea, how frequently and how much.

PATIENT INSTRUCTION SHEET 7(A) *contd*

Food for Days When You are Sick

It is important to continue to eat and drink. Small frequent meals may be easier to digest.

Suggested foods

- Sweetened jelly (not low cal)
- ice cream (1/2 cup)
- custard with sugar (1/2 cup)
- honey (3 teaspoons)
- sugar (1 tablespoon)
- sweetened ice block (one small or 90 ml)
- egg flip - sweetened (8 oz)
- tea or coffee + 4 teaspoons sugar
- milk (10 oz)
- Coke, lemonade or other sweetened soft drink (3/4 cup - not low cal)
- unsweetened tinned fruit (3/4 cup)
- orange juice (3/4 cup)
- apple juice (1/2 cup)
- pineapple juice (1/2 cup)
- orange (one medium)
- banana (one small)
- unflavoured yoghurt (100 g or 1/2 carton)
- flavoured (sweetened) yoghurt (200 g or one carton)
- broth or soup.

PATIENT INSTRUCTION SHEET 7(A) *contd*

Continuing Care

(1)   If the doctor prescribes antibiotics to treat the illness it is important to complete the full course.

(2)   Continue to test urine for ketones until they show clear for 24 hours.

(3)   Continue to test your blood glucose 2-4 hourly and record the results until you recover and then go back to your usual routine.

(4)   Go back to your usual food plan when you recover.

(5)   If your insulin has been increased during the illness decrease it again when you recover to avoid hypoglycaemia.

(6)   Consider writing down a medical history for quick reference in times of illness or in an emergency.

List:

- all the medications you are taking
- past illnesses
- blood group
- date of last tetanus and flu injection
- illnesses which run in the family.

This can be worn in an identification tag or be kept with your diabetes record book.

PATIENT INSTRUCTION SHEET 7(B): MANAGING YOUR DIABETES WHEN YOU ARE ILL: PATIENTS WITH TYPE 2 DIABETES

MANAGING YOUR DIABETES WHEN YOU ARE ILL

Illnesses (such as colds and flu) cause the body to make hormones which help the body fight the illness. These hormones usually also cause the blood glucose to go high. High blood glucose levels can lead to unpleasant symptoms like thirst, tiredness and passing a lot of urine.

By taking some simple precautions the minor illness can usually be treated at home.

What to Do

(1)   Continue to take your diabetes tablets. This is very important, because as we have said the blood glucose usually goes high. In severe illnesses or during an operation insulin injections may be needed until you recover.

(2)   Test your blood glucose every 2-4 hours. Write down the test results.

(3)   Continue to drink fluids or eat if possible (see recommended food list).

(4)   Read the labels on any medication you take to treat the illness because it may contain sugar, sugar substitutes or other ingredients which cause the blood glucose to go high.

(5)   Rest.

(6)   Keep the phone number of your doctor or diabetes educator beside the telephone.

PATIENT INSTRUCTION SHEET 7(B) *contd*

When to Call the Doctor

(1)   If you have diarrhoea and/or vomiting.

(2)   If the blood glucose continues to rise.

(3)   If you develop signs of dehydration (loss of skin tone, sunken eyes, dry mouth).

(4)   If the illness does not get better in 2-3 days.

(5)   If you feel you need advice.

What to Tell the Doctor When You Call

(1)   How long you have been sick.

(2)   What the blood glucose level is.

(3)   How long the blood glucose has been high.

(4)   How frequently you are passing urine and how much.

(5)   If you are thirsty, tired or have a temperature.

(6)   What medications you have taken to treat the illness.

(7)   If you have vomiting or diarrhoea, how frequently and how much.

PATIENT INSTRUCTION SHEET 7(B) *contd*

Food for Days When You are Sick

It is important to continue to eat and drink. Small frequent meals may be easier to digest.

Suggested foods

- sweetened jelly (not low cal)
- ice cream (1/2 cup)
- custard with sugar (1/2 cup)
- honey (3 teaspoons)
- sugar (1 tablespoon)
- sweetened ice block (one small or 90 ml)
- egg flip - sweetened (8 oz)
- tea or coffee + 4 teaspoons sugar
- milk (10 oz)
- Coke, lemonade or other sweetened soft drink (3/4 cup - not low cal)
- unsweetened tinned fruit (3/4 cup)
- orange juice (3/4 cup)
- apple juice (1/2 cup)
- pineapple juice (1/2 cup)
- orange (one medium)
- banana (one small)
- unflavoured yoghurt (100 g or 1/2 carton)
- flavoured (sweetened) yoghurt (200 g or one carton)
- broth or soup

PATIENT INSTRUCTION SHEET 7(B) *contd*

Continuing Care

(1)   If the doctor prescribes antibiotics to treat the illness it is important to complete the full course.

(2)   Continue to test your blood glucose 2-4 hourly and record the results until you recover and then go back to your usual routine.

(3)   Go back to your usual food plan when you recover.

(4)   Consider writing down a medical history for quick reference in times of illness or in an emergency.

List:

•   all the medications you are taking

•   past illnesses

•   blood group

•   date of last tetanus and flu injection

•   illnesses which run in the family.

This can be worn in an identification tag or be kept with your diabetes record book.

18.7   Further reading

CSL-NOVO Pty Ltd. *Diabetes Education Programme Training Notes.*

Green, W. & Simons-Morton, B. (1984) *Introduction to Health Education.* Macmillan, London.

Tupling, H. (1991) *You've Got to Get Through the Outside Layer.* David Ell Press, Sydney.

Chapter 19
Discharge Planning

19.1 Key points

- Commence early (on admission).
- Arrange follow-up care.
- Give contact telephone number.
- Ensure self-care knowledge is adequate.
- Ensure insulin and monitoring equipment is available.
- Ensure patient understands how and when to take medication.

A discharge plan must be established and conducted in a pro-active manner. It is important to build discharge planning into the initial assessment and patient care plan.

(1) Inform allied health professionals of admission on day one or two of admission (diabetes educator, dietitian, podiatrist, social worker).
(2) Ensure self-care status has been assessed so that the patient is capable of caring for his/her own diabetes and will be safe at home.
(3) Refer for domiciliary assessment early if indicated.

19.2 On day of discharge

(1) Ensure patient has necessary medications and supplies, syringes, monolets, diabetic record book and understands their use, and where to obtain future supplies.
(2) Ensure relevant follow-up appointments have been made, and a discharge letter has been written to the local doctor.
(3) If further tests are to be performed on an outpatient basis ensure patient has written instructions and understands what to do about medications and fasting.
(4) Ensure the patient has a contact telephone number for assistance if necessary.
(5) Ensure the patient knows about the services offered by the diabetic association.

19.2.1   Transfer to another hospital or nursing home

In addition to the usual information provided relating to nursing and medical management the nursing letter accompanying the patient should contain information about:

- Diet.
- Progress of diabetes education.
- Skills assessment for performing blood glucose testing and insulin administration.

Ensure transport has been arranged and that the family are aware of the discharge. Some nursing homes and special accommodation facilities may not have cared for people with diabetes in the past, or have done so on an infrequent basis. Diabetes education for the staff of the facility in this situation is desirable.

Chapter 20
Nursing Care in the Emergency and Outpatient Departments

20.1 Cross-references to other chapters

	Chapter
Minor surgery and medical procedures	13
Total parenteral nutrition	14
Continuous ambulatory peritoneal dialysis	14
Hypoglycaemia	8
Diabetic education and example patient instruction sheets	18
Hyperglycaemia/ketoacidosis	10
Hyperosmolar coma	10
Guidelines for outpatient stabilization onto insulin	9

20.2 The emergency department

Medical emergencies are a major source of morbidity and mortality for people with diabetes. The particular presenting problem may be unrelated to diabetes, however the existence of diabetes will usually affect metabolic control. Extra vigilance will be needed to reverse or limit the abnormalities arising as a consequence of altered glucose metabolism, due to stress, illness or trauma.

Diabetes related abnormalities frequently seen in the emergency department are:

- Myocardial infarct.
- Cerebrovascular accident.
- Severe hypoglycaemia.
- Infected/gangrenous feet.
- Hyperglycaemia.
- Ketoacidosis.
- Hyperosmolar coma.

Rapid effective therapy and effective nursing care increase the chance of a good recovery.

In urgent emergency situations clear short acting insulin is used.

20.2.1 Nursing responsibilities

(1) Carry out assessment and observations appropriate to the presenting complaint.
(2) Note patient identification tags.
(3) Enquire if the patient has diabetes.
(4) Record blood glucose.
(5) Record urine glucose and test for the presence of ketones.
(6) Ascertain time and dose of last diabetes medication.
(7) Ascertain time and amounts of last meal, especially the amount of carbohydrate consumed.
(8) Assess usual day-to-day diabetic control and the period of deteriorating control.
(9) Record any other medication, those prescribed by doctor and anything taken to relieve present complaint.
(10) Seek evidence of any underlying infection.
(11) Assess pain, severity, site, cause, and relieve appropriately.
(12) Consider the psychological aspects of the illness. Give full explanation to the patient and family.

- Blood glucose can be elevated by pain and anxiety.
- TPR and BP can also be affected by emotional stress.
- Reassure, rest the patient, repeat the TPR and BP.

(13) Avoid long delays in assessment if possible, and be aware of the possibility of a hypoglycaemic episode in diabetics on medication.
(14) Have appropriate carbohydrate available to treat promptly if hypoglycaemia does occur.

Hypoglycaemia may be masked by coma from other causes, some medications, and autonomic neuropathy.

(15) Assess diabetic knowledge and refer for further education if necessary.
(16) Ensure the patient knows when to take his/her next diabetes medication if discharged, especially if the dose has been adjusted, and that the patient understands the new dose.
(17) Arrange appropriate follow-up care.

20.3   The outpatient department

Patients may present to the outpatient department for routine appointments or for minor surgical or radiological procedures. They are usually basically well and mobile, although some may require a wheelchair, interpreter and/or guide dog assistance.

20.3.1   Nursing responsibilities

(1) Avoid long delays in seeing the doctor.
(2) Be aware of the possibility of hypoglycaemia and know how to recognize and treat it effectively. Have available at least one of the following:
  ● dry biscuits
  ● sandwiches
  ● tea/coffee, sugar
  ● orange juice
  ● glucose.
(3) Have blood glucose monitoring equipment available.
(4) Test urine of Type 1 diabetics for ketones if blood glucose is elevated.
(5) Ensure test results are available with the medical record.
(6) Ensure appropriate examination equipment is available:
  ● tendon hammer
  ● sterile pins
  ● ophthalmoscope
  ● tuning fork
  ● biothesiometer
  ● stethoscope
  ● eye chart
  ● midriatic drops.
(7) Ensure patient knows the location of toilets, other clinics, pharmacy.

Chapter 21
District Nursing and Domiciliary Care

21.1 Key points

- Establish communication link with referring agency.
- Assess patient before seeking medical advice.
- Ascertain if hyperglycaemia is a new occurrence.
- Seek cause for hypoglycaemia.

21.2 Introduction

Domiciliary care allows the provision of technical and professional care to acutely and chronically ill patients at home. The provision of the service will be influenced by the home environment. A nursing care plan should be drawn up in accordance with the medical management plan.

Maintaining people in their own homes is an important consideration of diabetic management. Visiting district and domiciliary nurses play an important role in this respect. They are often responsible for:

- Drawing up insulin.
- Administering insulin.
- Performing blood glucose tests.
- Assessing the general condition of the patient.
- Continuing the education of the patient.
- Attending to wound dressing.
- Attending to personal hygiene.

Making clinical decisions about the patient in the home situation without advice and support can be stressful and difficult. In addition, the home situation must be carefully assessed to ascertain how to obtain access to the home, and the correct address and telephone number. Other information (e.g. presence of dogs) should also be noted.

This chapter outlines the important diabetes-related information needed to gauge whether medical assessment is necessary.

21.3 How to obtain help

It is important for home care and domiciliary nursing bodies to establish open communication links with the referring agency:

- Hospital
- General practitioner

The referring agency should be the first point of contact for advice.

21.4 General points

(1) Ensure diabetes teaching is consistent with that of the diabetic unit.
(2) Before recommending equipment (meters, insulin pens, etc.) ensure the person will be able to use it and can afford it. Assess:
  - vision
  - manual dexterity
  - comprehension
  - and whether they understand the costs involved.
(3) Ensure the patient is enrolled in the National Diabetes Supply Scheme so that they can obtain syringes, lancets and test strips at the subsidized price (relevant only in Australia).

21.5 Diabetic problems commonly encountered in the home

(1) Finding an elevated blood glucose level.
(2) Hypoglycaemia.
(3) The patient has not taken their insulin/diabetes tablets and it is 11 AM or later.
(4) The patient who does not follow the diabetes management plan.
(5) Management of diabetic wounds (foot ulcers).
(6) Disposal of sharps (needles, monolets) in the home situation.
(7) How and where to obtain help/advice about specific patient problems.

21.6 Nursing actions

(1) Assess general clinical state (see Chapter 2).
(2) If the patient appears unwell, record:
  - temperature
  - pulse

- respiration
- blood pressure.

(3) Assess presence, location, duration and severity of any pain.
(4) Note nausea, diarrhoea and/or vomiting.
(5) Note presence of any symptoms of urinary tract infection:
- burning
- scalding
- itching.

(6) Assess state of hydration.
(7) Note time and dose of last diabetic medication.
(8) Note time and amount of last meal.
(9) Measure blood glucose level.

21.7 Interpreting the blood sugar level

To assess the diabetic status one must first ascertain whether the patient is in danger because of the blood glucose level. Ascertain:

- The present level.
- The usual blood glucose range.
- Why the blood glucose is outside the usual range.
- Where it is likely to go (up or down).

When ascertaining the blood glucose level check whether:

- The test was performed correctly.
- There was enough blood on the strip; if using a meter that the meter was calibrated and used correctly.
- The strips have exceeded the expiry date (See Chapter 4, monitoring 1: blood glucose).
- The patient has commenced any new medication which may alter the blood glucose level (see Chapter 6).

The patient may be in danger if the blood glucose level is:

- Low (hypoglycaemia <3 mmol/l).
- High (hyperglycaemia >17 mmol/l).

21.8 Hypoglycaemia

For more detailed information see Chapter 8.

(1) Treat according to the severity and time of occurrence of hypogly-caemia.

(2) Avoid overtreatment.
(3) Give rapidly absorbed glucose if symptomatic, e.g.:
- orange juice
- tea/coffee with sugar
- jelly beans.
(4) Give more slowly absorbed glucose if the hypoglycaemia is asymptomatic and there is some time before the next meal is due.
(5) Suggest they have their meal if it is due in half an hour.
(6) Ensure patient has recovered before leaving the home.
(7) Record incident; if severe seek medical assessment.

The next dose of medication is not usually withheld.

Discuss recognition and treatment of hypoglycaemia with patient and family.

21.9 Hyperglycaemia

For more detailed information see Chapter 10. Ascertain:

- How long the blood glucose level has been elevated.
- Whether the patient is unwell.
- Whether there are any symptoms of hyperglycaemia, e.g. polyuria, polydipsia, thirst or lethargy.
- Whether there are ketones present in the urine.

If moderate/heavy ketones are detected seek medical advice (this usually only occurs in Type 1 people).
  Check for any obvious source of infection:

- Urinary
- Foot ulcer
- Cold or flu

Counsel the patient about managing at home when unwell. (Patient information guidelines are shown in Chapter 18.) The important points are that the patient should:

- Continue to take insulin or OHAs.
- Maintain fluid and carbohydrate intake.
- Test and record blood glucose regularly, e.g. 2 to 4 hourly.

In addition:

(1) If the patient is insulin-dependent, they should test their urine for ketones every 4 hours.

(2) Maintain contact with the patient.
(3) Advise them to seek medical advice if vomiting and/or diarrhoea occurs, if the blood glucose continues to increase or if ketones develop in the urine.

21.10   The patient with chest pain

(1) Reassure the patient and family.
(2) Instruct the patient to stop current activity and to sit or lie down. Loosen tight clothing.
(3) Instruct patient to take anginine if prescribed by doctor.
(4) Assess the severity of the discomfort and the frequency of attacks.
(5) People with long-standing diabetes may have 'silent myocardial infarcts'. Complaints of vague chest discomfort should be investigated. The classic pain radiating into the jaw, arm and chest may be absent.
(6) Seek medical advice/ambulance service.
(7) Record BP.
(8) Discuss decreasing risk factors for cardiac disease (see Chapter 11).

21.11   The patient who has not taken their insulin or diabetes tablets and it is 11 AM or later

(1) Check blood glucose level.
(2) Ascertain why medication was omitted.
(3) Ascertain whether this is a regular occurrence.
(4) Ascertain whether they have eaten breakfast, and what they ate.

In general medication may need to be modified and the dose reduced. The amount will depend on the dose and types of insulin and the blood glucose level:

(1) Seek the advice of the referring agency.
(2) Document any medication adjustment.
(3) Have the order signed by the appropriate doctor within 24 hours.

If it is before 11 AM counsel the patient to check their blood glucose; if it is 6 mmol/l or above the patient should:

● Take usual medication dose and eat breakfast.
● Eat lunch within 3 to 4 hours then tea 3 to 4 hours after that.
● Have medication and breakfast at normal time the next day.

21.11.1 Follow-up visit

Ascertain whether:

- The patient followed advice.
- Hypo/hyperglycaemia occurred as a result of missed medication and modified dose.
- Further dietary counselling is necessary.

21.12 Managing diabetic foot ulcers at home

Diabetic foot ulcers are a common complication of diabetes and occur as a result of peripheral neuropathy and vascular changes (see Chapter 15).

21.12.1 On first visit

(1) Check treatment orders.
(2) Assess ulcer to obtain a baseline for future comparison:
- dimensions: width × depth
- type and quantity of discharge
- colour of surrounding tissue
- presence of oedema.
(3) Counsel patient to:
  (a) Rest with foot elevated as much as possible.
  (b) Protect foot:
- bed cradle (stiff cardboard or polystyrene box)
- appropriate footwear
- regular inspection.
  (c) Complete full course of antibiotics.
(4) Monitor blood glucose tests.

21.12.2 Further visits

(1) Perform the dressing according to prescribed orders. The dressing may be:
- dry
- occlusive
- or the wound may be cleaned and left open.
(2) Assess progress of the wound.
(3) If the wound deteriorates:
- take a swab for culture and sensitivity
- record TPR
- record blood glucose level
- refer for assessment.

If bandages are used ensure they are correctly applied and do not constrict the blood supply. People with neuropathy may not be able to tell if the bandage is too tight.

(1) Bandage from the foot upwards, even if the ulcer is on the leg.
(2) Do not put bandages or tape in a circular fashion around the toes.
(3) Never prick the toes to obtain a blood glucose test.

21.13 The patient who does not follow the management plan ('non-compliant'; see Chapter 17)

'Non-compliant' is a derogatory and negative term. There may well be good reasons why people do not follow prescribed treatment, including:

● A complicated regime that the patient does not understand.
● Treatment goals are those of the management team and not the patient.
● Inability to comply (patient may not have a refrigerator, low vision, loss of fine motor skills).
● Cultural and language differences.
● Economic factors – cost of supplies.
● Non-acceptance of diabetes and constraints imposed on lifestyle.
● Other concerns may outweigh those about diabetes.
● 'Burn out'.
● Learned helplessness.

Counselling, education and appropriate modification of health professional expectations may help. Behavioural changes may take years; patient, supportive health professionals and family assist the patient to eventually make some changes.

21.14 Disposal of sharps in the home situation

In the community the person with diabetes is responsible for the safe disposal of used needles and lancets. There are thousands of diabetes needles discarded every week, outside hospitals. All health professionals have a responsibility to promote the safe disposal of needles, syringes and lancets. The safe disposal of used needles, syringes and lancets should be an integral part of teaching injection technique, and blood glucose monitoring.

Ensure the patient understands what you mean by a 'sharp'.

21.14.1 Guidelines for handling and disposing of sharps at home

(1) Take care with sharps at all times.

(2) Store needles and monolets out of reach of children.

(3) Use a 'standards approved' container if possible (check with the local council about how to obtain one).

(4) Only recap your own syringe and lancet.

(5) Recapping of syringes and lancets is a good idea if an approved container is not available (e.g. at a restaurant).

(6) If testing blood glucose for family/friends always use a new monolet.

(7) Check arrangements for disposal of full containers with:
- your local Diabetes Association
- your local council.

(8) If an approved container is not available it is advisable to:
- recap needles and lancets
- place immediately into a puncture proof, unbreakable container, clearly labelled 'used sharps'
- keep the container out of the reach of children
- keep the lid tightly closed.

This information is based on guidelines developed by a subcommittee of Diabetes Australia.

21.15 Storage of insulin

Insulin should be stored in the fridge if possible; *it should not be frozen.* The vial in use can be stored at room temperature if protected from heat and light and should be used within one month of opening. Any unused insulin stored at room temperature should be discarded after one month.

If there is any change in appearance or consistency of the insulin, or if the expiry date is exceeded, discard the insulin.

21.16 Guidelines for premixing and storing insulin doses for domiciliary and district nursing services

21.16.1 General recommendations

Mixing and storage of insulin for periods of 24 hours or more may be necessary for the diabetic management of elderly patients, those with poor vision and those with limited hand mobility who live alone and where no other assistance is available.

The correct method of mixing short- and long-acting insulins are included in the Patient Instruction Sheets at the end of Chapter 18.

The proportions to be mixed are prescribed by the doctor to suit individual patient requirements. Neutral insulins such as Velosulin and Actrapid can be premixed with Isophane insulins, e.g. Protaphane, Isophane and Insulatard. They should not be premixed and stored with insulin zinc suspensions, e.g. Lente, Ultralente, Monotard.

21.16.2   Recommended guidelines

(1) Use insulin syringe only for drawing up insulin.
(2) The filled syringe should be stored:
  ● in the fridge if possible or in a cool dark place
  ● vertically or horizontally; they should not be stored with the needle pointing downwards which may cause clogging in the needle, preventing insulin being injected.
(3) Syringes should be rolled between the palms of the hands before administration to mix the contents.
(4) If the patient is on more than one injection per day the doses should be clearly understood by the patient.
(5) Injection technique should be assessed periodically to ensure insulin administration is accurate, especially in people with low vision and those with unexplained hyperglycaemia.
(6) One extra dose could be drawn up in case of emergencies provided the patient understands that it is not an extra dose of insulin.
(7) Monitor blood glucose when visiting the patient.
(8) Any concerns about control, mental state or accuracy of technique should be discussed with the relevant doctor.
(9) Signed and dated records of all advance doses of insulin (type, dose, frequency of administration) should be maintained. All blood glucose results and insulin doses should be recorded and accompany the patient to medical appointments.

If the patient has required a period in hospital, unused previously drawn up doses of insulin should be discarded. A new batch should be drawn up when the patient is discharged.

Appendix A
Associations Providing Services for People with Diabetes

A.1   Diabetic Associations

Diabetic associations have been established in most countries, including the UK (British Diabetic Association) and Australia (Diabetes Australia). Membership of these associations consists of lay people and health professionals who work together to develop management policies and educational material/programmes for the care of people with diabetes.

A.1.1   Diabetes Australia

Diabetes Australia (DA) is the national diabetes organization in Australia. It has branches in all states. A magazine, *Diabetes Conquest*, is produced quarterly. A national diabetes supply scheme (NDSS) is organized through Diabetes Australia and allows diabetic equipment (blood and urine test strips, syringes, meters) to be purchased at subsidized prices. People must enrol in the scheme, and a doctor's signature is required on the enrolment form. There is no cost to enrol. Supplies can be ordered and received by mail under this scheme. Insulin is not available through the NDSS scheme.

Address: Diabetes Australia
5/7 Phipps Place
Deakin 2600
ACT, Australia

A.1.2   British Diabetic Association

The British Diabetic Association (BDA) is the national diabetes organization in the UK, with 400 branches and groups. The BDA provides education, develops educational material and trains volunteers. A magazine, *Balance*, is produced six times each year.

Address: British Diabetic Association
10 Queen Anne Street
London W1M OBD
UK

Both associations can provide information about specific services available and whom to contact for advice or additional information. Both are active in promoting research into diabetes and fund raising activities to help finance diabetic research. Most of the reading material suitable for people with diabetes listed in Appendix C can be obtained from these associations.

A.1.3   USA

Similar services are provided in the USA by the American Diabetes Association. Enquiries can be directed to:

> American Diabetes Association
> 1660 Duke Street
> Alexandria VA 22314
> USA

A.2   Professional diabetes associations

Health professional groups with a particular interest in diabetes also work to ensure uniformity of diabetic information, a high standard of care and the professional development of their members. Such associations include:

- Australian Diabetes Educators Association.
- Australian Diabetes Society.
- American Association of Diabetes Educators.
- British Diabetic Association.
- Diabetes Educators International.
- European Association for the Study of Diabetes.
- Juvenile Diabetes Foundation.

A.3   International Diabetes Federation (IDF)

The IDF is an international federation of the national diabetes associations. An International Diabetes Federation Congress is held every three years in a different part of the world.

Address: International Diabetes Federation
International Association Centre
40 Rue Washington B-1050
Brussels, Belgium

00   322   538   4908

A.4   Other professional associations

Other professional associations have diabetic interest groups within their membership. They include:

- National heart foundations
- Kidney foundations
- Dietetics associations
- Podiatry associations

A.5   Pharmaceutical companies

Many of the pharmaceutical companies produce diabetic products and supply patient information leaflets. The major companies producing diabetic products are:

- Bayer Diagnostics
- Becton Dickinson
- Boehringer Mannheim
- Farmatalia Carlo Erba
- Hoechst Pharmaceuticals
- Novo Nordisk
- Servier Laboratories
- Terumo Corporation
- Wyeth

Addresses and telephone numbers can be found in the telephone directory, or from the diabetic association in your country.

Appendix B
Diabetes Reference Material for Nursing Staff

B.1 Reference texts

Galloway, J.A., Porvin, J.H. & Shuman, C.R. (eds) (1988) *Diabetes Mellitus*. Eli Lilly, Indianapolis.

Kozak, G.P. (ed.) (1992) *Clinical Diabetes Mellitus*. W.B. Saunders, Philadelphia.

Pickup, J.C. & Williams, G. (eds) (1991) *Textbook of Diabetes*. Blackwell Scientific Publications, Oxford.

Rifkin, H. & Porte, D. (eds) (1990) *Diabetes Mellitus, Theory and Practice*. Elsevier, New York.

Wilson, J. & Foster, D. (eds) (1985) *Williams Textbook of Endocrinology*. W.B. Saunders, Philadelphia.

B.2 Practical texts

Galloway, J. (ed.) (1988) *Diabetes Mellitus*. Eli Lilly, Indianapolis.

Krall, L.P. & Beasner, R.S. (1989) *Joslin Diabetes Manual*. Lea and Febiger, Philadelphia.

Taft, P. (ed.) (1985) *Diabetes Mellitus: A Guide to Treatment*. Ames Laboratories, Australia.

Williams, G. & Pickup, J. (eds) (1992) *Handbook of Diabetes*. Blackwell Scientific Publications, Oxford.

B.3 Recommended journals

The following journals are easy to read, contain clinically relevant articles and are available in most hospital libraries.

Diabetes Care (USA).
Diabetic Medicine (UK).
Diabetologia (Europe).
Practical Diabetes (UK).
The Diabetes Educator (USA).

Note: it is desirable to ensure that texts and articles are as current as possible so that information is not outdated.

Appendix C
Reading Material for People with Diabetes

Court, J. *Modern Living with Diabetes for all Ages*. Diabetes Australia.

Davidson, B. (1986) *New Diabetic Cookery*. Octopus, London.

Day, J., Brenchlay, S. & Redmond, S. *Living with Non-Insulin Dependent Diabetes*. Medikos, Sussex.

Day, J. *The Diabetes Handbook: Insulin Dependent Diabetes*. Thorsons Publishing, London.

Horn, B. (1990) *Living with Diabetes*. Houghton, Australia.

Krall, L. & Beaser, R.J. (1989) *Joslin Diabetes Manual*. Lea and Febiger, Philadelphia.

Moffit, P., Phillips, P. & Ayers, B (eds) (1991) *Diabetes and You, An Owner's Manual*. Diabetes Australia.

Roberts, C., McDonald, C. & Cox, M. (1990) *Eat and Enjoy*. Rene Gordon, Melbourne.

Sonksen, P., Fox, C. & Judd, S. *Diabetes at your Fingertips: The Comprehensive Diabetes Reference Book for the 1990s*. Class Publishing, London.

Stacy, P. & Borushek, A. (1986) *The Best Australian Cookbook for Diabetes and Weight Control*. Family Health Publications, Perth.

Diabetes Conquest, *Diabetes Forecast* and *Balance* are magazines for people with diabetes produced by the diabetic associations of Australia, the USA and the UK, respectively. They are available to people who become members of the relevant association.

Index